O G P L

Cardiovascular Problems

O G P L
OXFORD GENERAL PRACTICE LIBRARY

Cardiovascular Problems

Dr Nick Dunn

Senior Lecturer in Primary Medical Care,
University of Southampton and
General Practitioner,
New Milton, UK.

Dr Hazel Everitt

MRC Research Fellow and General Practitioner,
University of Southampton and Totton, UK.

and

Dr Chantal Simon

MRC Research Fellow and General Practitioner,
University of Southampton and
Totton, UK.

and Series Editor

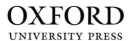

OXFORD
UNIVERSITY PRESS

OXFORD
UNIVERSITY PRESS

Great Clarendon Street, Oxford OX2 6DP

Oxford University Press is a department of the University of Oxford.
It furthers the University's objective of excellence in research, scholarship,
and education by publishing worldwide in

Oxford New York

Auckland Cape Town Dar es Salaam Hong Kong Karachi
Kuala Lumpur Madrid Melbourne Mexico City Nairobi
New Delhi Shanghai Taipei Toronto

With offices in

Argentina Austria Brazil Chile Czech Republic France Greece
Guatemala Hungary Italy Japan Poland Portugal Singapore
South Korea Switzerland Thailand Turkey Ukraine Vietnam

Oxford is a registered trade mark of Oxford University Press
in the UK and in certain other countries

Published in the United States
by Oxford University Press, Inc., New York

British Library Cataloguing in Publication Data
Data available

Library of Congress Cataloging in Publication Data
Data available

Typeset by Newgen Imaging Systems (P) Ltd., Chennai, India
Printed in Italy
on acid-free paper by
LegoPrint S.p.A.

ISBN 978–0–19–921571–3

10 9 8 7 6 5 4 3 2 1

Contents

Acknowledgements

This book would not have come into being without the support and drive of Peter Stevenson, Dominic Stow, Sara Chare, Emma Marchant and the rest of the team at Oxford University Press.

I would also like to thank Dr Kevin Fox and Dr Susan Connolly for their help in reviewing this book, Dr Francoise van Dorp for reviewing the sections relevant to paediatrics, Oliver Thompson for checking all the web links, and the authors of the Oxford Handbook of General Practice for allowing us to reproduce material.

All those involved in writing while working clinically, will be very aware that the real cost of such work is borne by families. I would like to dedicate this book to my wife Joanna, and my two children, Alice and Graham. Without you I would not have completed this book. You are truly the pride of my heart.

ND

Symbols and abbreviations

⚠	Warning
❗	Important note
☎	Controversial point
☎	Telephone number
💾	Website
📖	Cross reference to
±	With or without
↑	Increased/increasing
↓	Decreased/decreasing
→	Leading to
1°	Primary
2°	Secondary
♂	Male
♀	Female
≈	Approximately equal
~	Approximately
%	Percent(age)
≥	Greater than or equal to
≤	Less than or equal to
>	Greater than
<	Less than
+ve	Positive
-ve	Negative
o	Degrees
£	GMS contract payment available
C	Cochrane review
G	Guideline from major guideline producing body
N	NICE guidance
R	Randomized controlled trial in major journal
S	Systematic review in major journal
AA	Attendance allowance
AAA	Abdominal aortic aneurysm
A&E	Accident and emergency

ABPI	Ankle brachial pressure index
ACE	Angiotensin converting enzyme
AED	Automated external defibrillator
AF	Atrial fibrillation
Alk phos	Alkaline phosphatase
ALS	Advanced life support
ASD	Atrial septal defect
AST	Aspartate amino transferase
AV	Atrioventricular
A-V	Arterio-venous
bd	Twice daily
BHF	British Heart Foundation
BHS	British Hypertension Society
BJGP	British Journal of General Practice
BLS	Basic life support
BMA	British Medical Association
BMD	Bone mineral density
BMI	Body mass index
BMJ	British Medical Journal
BNF	British National Formulary
BP	Blood pressure
bpm	Beats per minute
Ca^{2+}	Calcium
CABG	Coronary artery bypass graft
CCF	Congestive cardiac failure
CHD	Coronary heart disease
CK	Creatine kinase
cm	Centimetre(s)
CNS	Central nervous system
COC	Combined oral contraceptive
COPD	Chronic obstructive pulmonary disease
Cr	Creatinine
CRP	C-reactive protein
CSM	Committee on Safety in Medicine
CT	Computed tomography scan
CVA	Stroke
CVD	Cardiovascular disease
CPR	Cardiopulmonary resuscitation
CXR	Chest X-ray
d.	Day(s)

DC	Direct current
DEXA	Dual energy X-ray absorptionometry
DLA	Disability Living Allowance
DM	Diabetes mellitus
DN	District nurse
DoH	Department of Health
DTB	Drugs and Therapeutic Bulletin
DVLA	Driver and Vehicle Licensing Authority
DVT	Deep vein thrombosis
Echo	Echocardiogram
ECG	Electrocardiograph
e.g.	For example
ESR	Erythrocyte sedimentation rate
etc.	Et cetera
FBC	Full blood count
FH	Family history
GGT or γGT	Gamma glutmyl transferase
GI	Gastrointestinal
GMS	General Medical Services
GP	General Practitioner
GTN	Glyceryl trinitrate
GU	Genitourinary
h.	Hour(s)
HDL	High density lipoprotein
HGV	Heavy goods vehicle
HOCM	Hypertrophic obstructive cardiomyopathy
HRT	Hormone replacement therapy
IHD	Ischaemic heart disease
IM	Intramuscular
INR	International normalization ratio
IS	Income support
IT	Information technology
IUCD	Intrauterine contraceptive device
IUGR	Intrauterine growth retardation
ISMO	Isosorbide mononitrate
IV	Intravenous
J	Joules
JAMA	Journal of the American Medical Association
JSA	Jobseekers Allowance
JVP	Jugular venous pressure

K+	Potassium
kg	Kilogram(s)
LBBB	Left bundle branch block
LDH	Lactate dehydrogenase
LDL	Low density lipoprotein
LFTs	Liver function tests
LMWH	Low molecular weight heparin
LOC	Loss of consciousness
LVF	Left ventricular failure
LVH	Left ventricular hypertrophy
M, C&S	Microscopy, culture and sensitivities
m.	Metres
mcgm.	Micrograms
mg	Milligrams
Mg^{2+}	Magnesium
MI	Myocardial infarct
min.	Minutes
mmHg	Millimetres of mercury
MND	Motor neurone disease
mo.	Month(s)
MoD	Ministry of Defence
MRI	Magnetic resonance imaging
MS	Multiple sclerosis
MSU	Mid-stream urine
NEJM	New England Journal of Medicine
NHS	National Health Service
NICE	National Institute for Clinical Excellence
NSAID	Non-steroidal anti-inflammatory drug
NSF	National Service Framework
O_2	Oxygen
od	Once daily
OT	Occupational therapy/ therapist
OTC	Over the counter
OUP	Oxford University Press
p.	Page number
PALS	Paediatric advanced life support
PAN	Polyarteritis nodosum
PBLS	Paediatric basic life support
PCO	Primary Care Organization
PDA	Patent ductus arteriosus

PE	Pulmonary embolus
Physio	Physiotherapy
PMH	Past medical history
PMR	Polymyalgia rheumatica
PMS	Personal Medical Services
PND	Paroxysmal nocturnal dyspnoea
po	Oral
PO_4	Phosphate
PPI	Proton pump inhibitor
prn	As needed
PSV	Public service vehicle
RBC	Red blood cell
RBBB	Right bundle branch block
RCT	Randomized controlled trial
RVF	Right ventricular failure
RVH	Right ventricular hypertrophy
s. or sec.	Second (s)
SAH	Subarachnoid haemorrhage
SBE	Subacute bacterial endocarditis
SIGN	Scottish Intercollegiate Guidelines Network
SLE	Systemic lupus erythematosis
s/ling	Sub-lingual
SVC	Superior vena cava
SVT	Supraventricular tachycardia
TB	Tuberculosis
TCA	Tricyclic antidepressant
tds	Three times a day
TFTs	Thyroid function tests
TG	Triglyceride
TIA	Transient ischaemic attack
TSH	Thyroid stimulating hormone
u.	Unit(s)
U&E	Urea and electrolytes
UC	Ulcerative colitis
UK	United Kingdom
USS	Ultrasound scan
UTI	Urinary tract infection
VDU	Visual display unit
VF	Ventricular fibrillation
VSD	Ventricular septal defect

VT	Ventricular tachycardia
WHO	World Health Organization
wk.	Week(s)
WPW	Wolff-Parkinson-White
y.	Year(s)

Chapter 1

Resuscitation in primary care

1

Managing a resuscitation attempt outside hospital

Resuscitation equipment: See Table 1.1
- Resuscitation equipment is used relatively infrequently. Staff must know where to find equipment and be trained to use the equipment to a level appropriate to the individual's expected role.
- Each practice should have a named individual with responsibility for checking the state of readiness of all resuscitation drugs and equipment, on a regular basis, ideally once a week. In common with drugs, disposable items like the adhesive electrodes have a finite shelf life and will require replacement from time to time if unused.

Training: Training and practice are necessary to acquire skill in resuscitation techniques. Resuscitation skills decline rapidly and updates and retraining using manikins are necessary every 6–12mo. to maintain adequate skill levels. Level of resuscitation skill needed by different members of the primary health care team differs according to the individual's role:
- All those in direct contact with patients should be trained in basic life support (BLS) and related resuscitation skills e.g. the recovery position
- Doctors, nurses and other paramedical workers (e.g. physiotherapists) should be able to use an automatic external defibrillator (AED). Other personnel (e.g. receptionists) may also be trained to use an AED.

Basic life support: Adults – 🕮 p.6; Children – 🕮 p.12

The recovery position: 🕮 p.18

Automatic external defibrillators: Adults – 🕮 p.7; Children – 🕮 p.13

Advanced life support: Adults – 🕮 p.11; Children – 🕮 p.17

Performance management:
- Accurate records of all resuscitation attempts and electronic data stored by most AEDs during a resuscitation attempt should be kept for audit, training and medico-legal reasons.
- The responsibility for this rests with the most senior member of the practice team involved.
- Process and outcome of all resuscitation attempts should be audited – at practice and PCO level – to allow deficiencies to be addressed, and examples of good practice to be shared.

Essential reading
Resuscitation Council (UK) Cardiopulmonary resuscitation guidance for clinical practice and training in Primary Care (2001) 🖥 www.resus.org.uk

GP Notes: ⚠ Importance of resuscitation training

- Ventricular fibrillation complicating acute MI is the most common cause of cardiac arrest that members of the primary health care team will encounter.
- Success is greatest when the event is witnessed and attempted defibrillation is performed with the minimum of delay.
- It is unacceptable for patients who sustain a cardiopulmonary arrest to await the arrival of the ambulance service before basic resuscitation is performed and a defibrillator is available.

Table 1.1 Resuscitation equipment needed

Equipment	Notes
Defibrillator with electrodes and razor	An automated external defibrillator should be available wherever and whenever sick patients are seen. Regular maintenance is needed even if the machine is not used. After the machine is used the manufacturers instructions should be followed to return it to a state of readiness with minimum delay.
Pocket mask with 1-way valve	All personnel should be trained to use one.
Oro-pharyngeal airway	Suitable for use by those appropriately trained. Keep a range of sizes available.
Oxygen and mask with reservoir bag	Should be available wherever possible. Oxygen cylinders need regular maintenance—follow national safety standards.
Suction	Simple, mechanical, portable, hand-held suction devices are recommended.
Drugs	Epinephrine/adrenaline—1mg IV Atropine—3mg IV (give once only) – for bradycardia, asystole and pulseless electrical activity Amiodarone—300mg IV—for VF resistant to defibrillation Naloxone—for suspected cases of respiratory arrest due to opiate overdose ⚠ There is no evidence for the use of alkalizing agents, buffers or calcium salts before hospitalization. Drugs should be given by the intravenous route, preferably through a catheter placed in a large vein, for example in the antecubital fossa, and flushed in with a bolus of IV fluid. Many drugs may be given via the bronchial route if a tracheal tube is in place and it is impossible to establish IV/IO acccess; for epinephrine/adrenaline and atropine the dose is double the IV dose.
Other	Saline flush, gloves, syringes and needles, IV cannulae, IV fluids, sharps box, scissors, tape

Ethical issues

- It is essential to identify individuals in whom cardiopulmonary arrest is a terminal event and where resuscitation is inappropriate.
- Overall responsibility for a 'do not attempt to resuscitate (DNAR)' decision rests with the doctor in charge of the patient's care.
- Seek opinions of other members of the medical and nursing team, the patient and any relatives in reaching a DNAR decision.
- Record the patient should not be resuscitated in the notes, the reasons for that decision and what the relatives have been told.
- Ensure all members of the multidisciplinary team involved with the patient's care are aware of the decision and record it in their notes.
- Review the decision not to attempt resuscitation regularly in the light of the patient's condition.

Essential reading

BMA, RCN and Resuscitation Council (UK) Decisions relating to cardiopulmonary resuscitation (2001) ▣ www.resus.org.uk

GMS contract		
Education 1	There is a record of all practice-employed clinical staff having attended training/updating in basic life support skills in the preceding 18mo.	4 points
Education 5	There is a record of all practice-employed staff having attended training/updating in basic life support skills in the preceding 36mo.	3 points
Education 7	Practice has undertaken ≥12 significant event reviews in the past 3y. which could include any deaths occurring in the practice premises	Total of 4 points for 12 significant event reviews
Management 7	The practice has systems in place to ensure regular and appropriate inspection, calibration, maintenance and replacement of equipment including: • A defined responsible person • Clear recording • Systematic pre-planned schedules • Reporting of faults	3 points
Medicines 3	There is a system for checking the expiry dates of emergency drugs on at least an annual basis	2 points

Basic adult life support

Basic paediatric life support: 📖 p.13

Basic adult life support (BLS): is a holding operation–sustaining life until help arrives. BLS should be started as soon as the arrest is detected – outcome is less good the longer the delay.

1. Danger: Ensure safety of rescuer and patient

2. Response: Check the patient for any response
- Is he **A**lert? Yes/No
- Does he respond to **V**ocal stimuli? Yes/No
- Does he respond to a **P**ainful stimulus (pinching the lower part of the nasal septum)? Yes/No
- Is the patient **U**nconscious? Yes/No

If he responds by answering or moving: Don't move the patient unless in danger. Get help. Reassess regularly.

If he does not respond: Shout for help; turn the patient on to his back.

3. Airway: Open the airway – place one hand on the patient's forehead and tilt his head back. With fingertips under the point of the patient's chin, lift the chin to open the airway.

⚠ Try to avoid head tilt if trauma to the neck is suspected

4. Breathing: With airway open, look, listen and feel for breathing for no more than 10 sec. – look for chest movement, listen at the victim's mouth for breath sounds, feel for air on your cheek.

If breathing normally: Turn the patient into the recovery position (📖 p.18), get help and check for continued breathing

If not breathing or only making occasional gasps/weak attempts at breathing: Get help then start chest compressions.

ⓘ In the first few minutes after cardiac arrest, a victim may be barely breathing, or taking infrequent, noisy, gasps. Don't confuse this with normal breathing. If you have any doubt whether breathing is normal, act as if it is not normal.

5. Circulation: Start chest compressions if not breathing:
- Kneel by the side of the victim and place the heel of 1 hand in the centre of the victim's chest. Place the heel of your other hand on top of the first hand. Interlock the fingers of your hands and ensure that pressure is not applied over the victim's ribs. Don't apply any pressure over the upper abdomen or the bottom end of the bony sternum
- Position yourself vertically above the victim's chest and, with arms straight, press down on the sternum 4–5cm
- After each compression, release all the pressure on the chest without losing contact between your hands and the sternum. Compression and release should take an equal amount of time
- Repeat at a rate of ~100x/min.

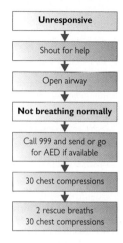

Figure 1.1 Basic life support (BLS) algorithm

Unresponsive

↓

Shout for help

↓

Open airway

↓

Not breathing normally

↓

Call 999 and send or go for AED if available

↓

30 chest compressions

↓

2 rescue breaths
30 chest compressions

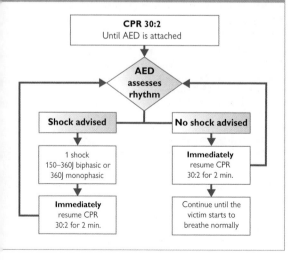

Figure 1.2 Automated external defibrillator (AED) algorithm

CPR 30:2
Until AED is attached

↓

AED assesses rhythm

Shock advised → **No shock advised**

↓

1 shock
150–360J biphasic or
360J monophasic

↓

Immediately
resume CPR
30:2 for 2 min.

Immediately
resume CPR
30:2 for 2 min.

↓

Continue until the
victim starts to
breathe normally

Figures 1.1 and 1.2 are reproduced from the Resuscitation Guidelines (2005) with permission
🖳 www.resus.org.uk

6. Combine chest compression with rescue breaths:

- After 30 compressions open the airway using head tilt and chin lift
- Pinch the soft part of the victim's nose closed, using the index finger and thumb of your hand on his forehead. Allow the victim's mouth to open, but maintain chin lift.
- Give a rescue breath – take a normal breath and place your lips around the victim's mouth (mouth-to-nose technique is an alternative) making sure that you have a good seal. Blow steadily into his mouth for ~1sec. whilst watching for the chest to rise
- Maintaining head tilt and chin lift, take your mouth away from the victim and watch for the chest to fall as air comes out.
- Take another normal breath and blow into the victim's mouth again to give a total of 2 effective rescue breaths. Then return your hands without delay to the correct position on the sternum and give a further 30 chest compressions.
- Continue chest compressions and rescue breaths in a ratio of 30:2.

⚠ If rescue breaths don't make the chest rise:

- Check the victim's mouth and remove any visible obstruction
- Recheck that there is adequate head tilt and chin lift
- Don't attempt >2 breaths each time before returning to chest compressions

Chest-compression-only CPR: If you are unable or unwilling to give rescue breaths, give continuous chest compressions only at a rate of 100/min.

> ⚠ Only stop to recheck the victim if the patient makes a movement or takes a spontaneous breath; otherwise resuscitation should not be interrupted

Use of automated external defibrillators (AEDs) in adults:

Program AEDs to deliver a single shock followed by a pause of 2min for the immediate resumption of CPR.

If a patient arrests: Start CPR according to the guidelines for basic life support.

As soon as the AED arrives:

- Switch on the AED and attach the electrode pads. If >1 rescuer is present, continue CPR whilst this is done. (Some AEDs automatically switch on when the AED lid is opened).
  - Place one AED pad to the right of the sternum, below the clavicle.
  - Place the other pad in the mid-axillary line with its long axis vertical
- Follow the voice / visual prompts. Ensure nobody touches the victim whilst the AED is analysing the rhythm.

If a shock is indicated: Ensure nobody touches the victim. Push the shock button as directed (fully-automatic AEDs deliver the shock automatically). Immediately resume CPR and continue to follow the prompts.

If no shock is indicated: Immediately resume CPR and continue to follow the prompts.

Use of AEDs in children: 📖 p.14

GP Notes:

When to go for assistance: It is vital for rescuers to get assistance as quickly as possible. If you are the only rescuer, and the victim is an adult, call for assistance before starting CPR.

When >1 rescuer is available:
- One should start resuscitation while another goes for assistance
- Another should take over CPR every 2 min. to prevent fatigue. Ensure minimum of delay during changeover of rescuers.

Duration of resuscitation: Continue resuscitation until:
- Qualified help arrives and takes over
- The victim starts breathing normally
- You become exhausted

Automated external defibrillators (AEDs):
- Modern automated external defibrillators have simplified the process of defibrillation considerably.
- The use of such machines should be within the capabilities of all medical and nursing staff working in the community so ALL practices should have an AED.
- Increasingly trained lay persons are successfully employing AEDs and it is quite appropriate for reception, administrative and secretarial staff to be trained in their use.

Pad position: Place 1 pad to the right of the sternum below the clavicle. Place the other pad vertically in the midaxillary line approximately level with the v6 ECG electrode position or female breast (though clear of any breast tissue).

GMS contract

Education 1	There is a record of all practice-employed clinical staff having attendedtraining/updating in basic life support skills in the preceding 18 mo.	4 points
Education 5	There is a record of all practice em-ployed staff having attended training/ updating in basic life support skills in the preceding 36 mo.	3 points

Further reading
Resuscitation Council (UK) Resuscitation guidelines (2005)
www.resus.org.uk

Adult advanced life support

- 3 stages:
  - Revive the patient using basic life support (📖 p.6). Basic life support should be started if there is any delay in obtaining a defibrillator, but must not delay shock delivery.
  - Restore spontaneous cardiac output, using an automatic external defibrillator (📖 p.7) or manual defibrillator.
  - Review possible causes for cardiac arrest and take further action as needed

Precordial thump: Appropriate if the arrest is witnessed and and a defibrillator is not to hand – may dislodge a pulmonary embolus or 'jerk' the heart back into sinus rhythm. Use the ulnar edge of a tightly clenched fist and deliver a sharp impact to the lower ½ of the sternum from a height of ~20cm then immediately retract the fist.

VF/VT arrest:

- Attempt defibrillation (1 shock 150–200J biphasic or 360J monophasic)
- Immediately resume chest compressions (30:2) without reassessing rhythm or feeling for the pulse. Continue CPR for 2min. then pause briefly to check the monitor
- If VT/VF persists give a 2nd shock (150–360J biphasic or 360J monophasic), continue CPR for 2min. then pause briefly to check the monitor
- If VF/VT persists give adrenaline (epinephrine) 1mg IV (or intraosseously if IV access cannot be attained) followed immediately by a 3rd shock (150–360J biphasic or 360J monophasic). Resume CPR immediately and continue for 2min. then pause briefly to check the monitor.
- If VF/VT persists give amiodarone 300mg IV (lidocaine 1mg/kg is an alternative if amiodarone isn't available) followed immediately by a 4th shock (150–360J biphasic or 360J monophasic). Resume CPR immediately and continue for 2min.
- Give adrenaline (epinephrine) 1mg IV immediately before alternate shocks (i.e. approximately every 3–5min).
- Give a further shock after each 2min period of CPR and after confirming that VF/VT persists.

Non-VT/VF arrest:

- Start CPR 30:2. Without stopping CPR, check that the leads are attached correctly.
- Give adrenaline (epinephrine) 1mg IV as soon as IV access is achieved.
- If asystole or pulseless electrical activity with rate <60 beats/min., give atropine 3mg IV (once only).
- Continue CPR 30:2 until the airway is secured, then continue chest compression without pausing during ventilation.
- Recheck the rhythm after 2min and proceed accordingly.
- Give adrenaline (epinephrine) 1mg IV every 3–5min (alternate loops)

Fine VF: Fine VF difficult to distinguish from asystole is very unlikely to be shocked successfully into a perfusing rhythm. Continuing good quality CPR may improve the amplitude and frequency of the VF and improve the chance of successful defibrillation to a perfusing rhythm.

Organised electrical activity: If organized electrical activity is seen during the brief pause in compressions, check for a pulse.
● If a pulse is present, start post-resuscitation care (📖 p.18)
● If no pulse, continue CPR and follow the non-shockable algorithm.

Defibrillator pad position: 📖 p.9

Further reading

Resuscitation Council (UK) *Resuscitation guidelines* (2005)
🖥 www.resus.org.uk

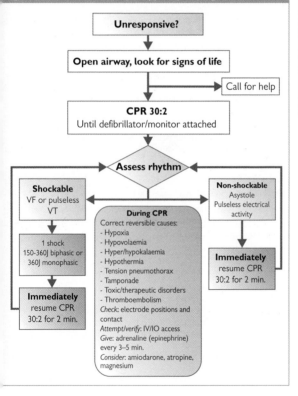

Figure 1.3 Adult advanced life support (ALS) algorithm

Unresponsive?

Open airway, look for signs of life

Call for help

CPR 30:2
Until defibrillator/monitor attached

◆ **Assess rhythm** ◆

Shockable
VF or pulseless VT

Non-shockable
Asystole
Pulseless electrical activity

During CPR
Correct reversible causes:
- Hypoxia
- Hypovolaemia
- Hyper/hypokalaemia
- Hypothermia
- Tension pneumothorax
- Tamponade
- Toxic/therapeutic disorders
- Thromboembolism
Check: electrode positions and contact
Attempt/verify: IV/IO access
Give: adrenaline (epinephrine) every 3–5 min.
Consider: amiodarone, atropine, magnesium

1 shock
150-360J biphasic or 360J monophasic

Immediately
resume CPR
30:2 for 2 min.

Immediately
resume CPR
30:2 for 2 min.

Figure 1.3 is reproduced from Resuscitation Guidelines (2005) with permission. Full version available from 🖥 www.resus.org.uk

Basic paediatric life support

Basic life support is a holding operation – sustaining life until help arrives.

Danger: Ensure safety of rescuer and patient

Response: Check the child for any response
- Is he **A**lert?
- Does he respond to **V**ocal stimuli?
- Does he respond to **P**ainful stimuli (pinch lower part of nasal septum)?
- Is he **U**nconscious?

If he responds by answering or moving: Don't move the child unless in danger. Get help. Reassess regularly.

If he does not respond: Shout for help. Assess airway (below).

Airway: Open the airway. Don't move the child from the position in which you found him unless you have to:
- Gently tilt the head back – with your hand on the child's forehead
- Lift the chin – with your fingertips under the point of the child's chin

If unsuccessful:
- Try jaw thrust – place the first 2 fingers of each hand behind each side of the child's jaw bone and push the jaw forward.
- Try lifting the chin or jaw thrust after carefully turning the child onto his back

⚠ Avoid head tilt as much as possible if trauma to the neck is suspected

Breathing: Look, listen and feel for breathing (maximum 10sec.)

If breathing normally: Turn the child carefully into the recovery position (📖 p.18) if unconscious, and check for continued breathing

If not breathing or making agonal gasps (infrequent irregular breaths):
- Carefully turn the child onto his back and remove any obvious airway obstruction.
- Give 5 initial rescue breaths – note any gag or cough response

Technique for rescue breaths:
- Ensure head tilt (neutral position for children<1y.) and chin lift.
- If age ≥1y., pinch the soft part of the child's nose closed with the index finger and thumb of the hand which is on his forehead. Open the child's mouth a little, but maintain the chin upwards.
- Take a breath and place your lips around the child's mouth (mouth and nose if <1y.*), ensuring you have a good seal. Blow steadily into the child's airway over ~1–1.5 sec watching for chest rise.
- Maintaining head tilt and chin lift, take your mouth away and watch for the chest to fall as air comes out.
- Take another breath and repeat this sequence 5 times.

❗ If you have difficulty achieving an effective breath, consider airway obstruction – 📖 p.14

---

* If the nose and mouth can't both be covered place your lips around the mouth alone as for an older child, or nose alone and close the child's lips to prevent air escape.

Figure 1.4 Paediatric basic life support (PBLS) algorithm

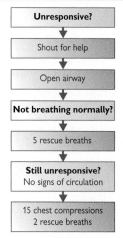

Unresponsive?

↓

Shout for help

↓

Open airway

↓

Not breathing normally?

↓

5 rescue breaths

↓

Still unresponsive?
No signs of circulation

↓

15 chest compressions
2 rescue breaths

After 1 minute call for help then continue CPR

Figure 1.5 Automated external defibrillator (AED) algorithm

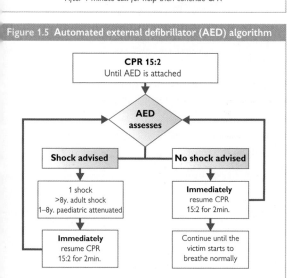

CPR 15:2
Until AED is attached

↓

AED assesses

Shock advised | **No shock advised**

1 shock
>8y. adult shock
1–8y. paediatric attenuated

Immediately
resume CPR
15:2 for 2min.

Immediately
resume CPR
15:2 for 2min.

Continue until the
victim starts to
breathe normally

Figures 1.4 and 1.5 are reproduced from *Resuscitation Guidelines* (2005) with permission. Full version available from 🖳 www.resus.org.uk

If the child is **UNCONSCIOUS** and foreign body airways obstruction is a possibility: ⊙ Don't leave the child
- Place on a firm, flat surface – call out/send for help if not arrived
- Open the mouth and look for any obvious object. If one is seen, make an attempt to remove it with a single finger sweep.
- *Rescue breaths:* Open the airway and attempt 5 rescue breaths. Assess effectiveness of each breath – if a breath doesn't make the chest rise, reposition the head before making the next attempt.
- If there is no response to the rescue breaths, proceed immediately to chest compression – regardless of whether the breaths were successful. Follow the PBLS sequence for 1 minute before summoning help if not already there.

Circulation (signs of life): Check (maximum 10sec.) for:
- Any movement, coughing or normal breathing (not agonal gasps)
- Pulse – child ≥1y. carotid pulse; child <1y. brachial pulse

If circulation is present: Continue rescue breathing until the child starts breathing effectively on his own. Turn the child into the recovery position (📖 p.18) if unconscious, and reassess frequently.

If circulation is absent: or slow pulse (<60 beats/min.) with poor perfusion, or you are not sure:
- Give 15 chest compressions. Then give 2 rescue breaths followed by 15 further chest compressions.
- Continue the cycle of 2 breaths followed by 15 chest compressions.

⊙ Lone rescuers may use a ratio of 30 compressions : 2 rescue breaths

Technique for chest compressions: Compress the sternum 1 finger's breadth above the xiphisternum by $\sim^1/_3$ of the depth of the chest. Release the pressure then repeat at a rate of ~100 compressions/min.
- Children <1y. with a lone rescuer – use the tips of 2 fingers
- Children <1y. with ≥2 rescuers – place both thumbs flat on the lower $^1/_3$ of the sternum with tips pointing towards the child's head and encircle the lower part of the child's ribcage with the tips of the fingers supporting the infant's back. Press down with both thumbs.
- Children >1y. – place the heel of 1 hand over the lower $^1/_3$ of the sternum. Lift the fingers. Position yourself vertically above the chest with arm straight, and push downwards. For larger children use both hands with fingers interlocked to achieve satisfactory compressions.

⚠ Stop to recheck for signs of a circulation only if the child moves or takes a spontaneous breath – otherwise continue uninterrupted

Use of automated external defibrillators (AEDs) in children:
- Children >8y.: Use the standard adult AED
- Children aged 1–8y.: Paediatric pads or a paediatric mode should be used if available – if not, use the adult AED as it is.
- Children <1y.: AED use is currently not advised.

If a patient arrests: Start CPR according to the guidelines for PBLS

As soon as the AED arrives:

- Switch on the AED and attach the electrode pads. If >1rescuer is present, continue CPR whilst this is done. (Some AEDs automatically switch on when the AED lid is opened).
  - Place one AED pad to the right of the sternum, below the clavicle.
  - Place the other pad in the mid-axillary line with its long axis vertical
- Follow the voice / visual prompts. Ensure nobody touches the victim whilst the AED is analysing the rhythm.

If a shock is indicated: Ensure nobody touches the victim. Push the shock button as directed (fully-automatic AEDs deliver the shock automatically). Immediately resume CPR and continue to follow the prompts.

If no shock is indicated: Immediately resume CPR and continue to follow the prompts.

GP Notes:

When to go for assistance: It is vital for rescuers to get assistance as quickly as possible when a child collapses.

When >1 rescuer is available: One should start resuscitation while another rescuer goes for assistance

Lone rescuer: Perform resuscitation for *1 minute* before going for assistance (and consider taking a young child/infant with you to minimize interruption in CPR). The only exception to this is a *witnessed sudden* collapse - as in this case cardiac arrest is likely to be due to arrhythmia and the child may need defibrillation so seek help immediately.

Duration of resuscitation: Continue resuscitation until:
- child shows signs of life (spontaneous respiration, pulse, movement)
- further qualified help arrives
- you become exhausted

Cervical spine injury:
- If spinal cord injury is suspected (e.g. if the victim has sustained a fall, been struck on the head or neck, or has been rescued after diving into shallow water) take particular care during handling and resuscitation to maintain alignment of the head, neck and chest in the neutral position.
- A spinal board and/or cervical collar should be used if available.

GMS contract

Education 1	There is a record of all practice-employed clinical staff having attended training/updating in basic life support skills in the preceding 18 mo.	4 points
Education 5	There is a record of all practice employed staff having attended training/ updating in basic life support skills in the preceding 36 mo.	3 points

Further information
Resuscitation Council (UK) Resuscitation guidelines (2005)
⊞ www.resus.org.uk

15

Advanced paediatric life support

Cardiac arrest in children is rare. Unless there is underlying heart disease, it is usually a consequence of respiratory arrest which results in asystole or pulseless electrical activity and has poor prognosis. Good airway management and providing high flow oxygen for very sick children is therefore important in preventing cardiac arrest.

Basic paediatric life support: Follow the algorithm on 📖 p.13

Unable to ventilate? Consider foreign body in the airway and initiate airway obstruction sequence – 📖 p.14

Checking the pulse:
- *Child* – feel for the carotid pulse in the neck
- *Infant* – feel for the brachial pulse on the inner aspect of the upper arm.

Once the airway is protected: If the aiway is protected by tracheal intubation, continue chest compression without pausing for ventilation. Provide ventilation at a rate of 10/min and compression at 100/min.

When circulation is restored, ventilate the child at a rate of 12–20 breaths/min.

Adrenaline (epinephrine) dose:
- Intravenous or interosseous (IO) access – 10 mcgm/kg adrenaline (0.1ml/kg of 1:10,000 solution)
- If circulatory access is not present, and can't be quickly obtained, but the child has a tracheal tube in place, consider giving adrenaline 100mcgm/kg via the tracheal tube (1ml/kg of 1:10,000 or 0.1ml/kg of 1:1,000 solution).This is the least satisfactory route of administration.

⚠ Don't give 1:1000 adrenaline IV or IO

VF/Pulseless VT: Less common in paediatric life support.
- Defibrillation:
  - Give 1 shock of 4J/kg or
  - If using an AED for a child of 1–8 y. deliver a paediatric attenuated adult shock energy.
  - If using an AED for a child >8 y. use the adult shock energy
- For VF/pulseless VT persisting after the 3rd shock, try amiodarone 5mg/kg diluted in 5% dextrose.

Bradycardia: When bradycardia is unresponsive to improved ventilation and circulatory support, try atropine 20mcgm/kg (maximum dose 600mcgm; minimum dose 100mcgm)

Magnesium: Magnesium treatment is indicated in children with documented hypomagnesemia or with polymorphic VT ('torsade de pointes'), regardless of cause. Give IV magnesium sulphate over several minutes at a dose of 25–50 mg/kg (to a maximum of 2g).

Intravenous fluids: In situations where the cardiac arrest has resulted from circulatory failure, a standard (20ml/kg) bolus of crystalloid fluid should be given if there is no response to the initial dose of epinephrine.

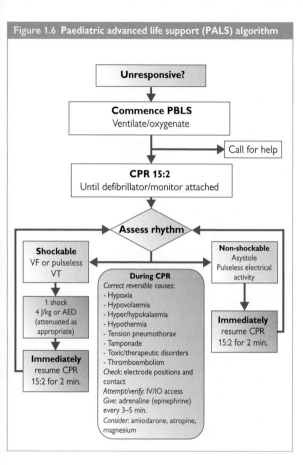

Figure 1.6 Paediatric advanced life support (PALS) algorithm

Unresponsive?

Commence PBLS
Ventilate/oxygenate

Call for help

CPR 15:2
Until defibrillator/monitor attached

Assess rhythm

Shockable
VF or pulseless VT

Non-shockable
Asystole
Pulseless electrical activity

1 shock
4 J/kg or AED
(attenuated as appropriate)

Immediately
resume CPR
15:2 for 2 min.

Immediately
resume CPR
15:2 for 2 min.

During CPR
Correct reversible causes:
- Hypoxia
- Hypovolaemia
- Hyper/hypokalaemia
- Hypothermia
- Tension pneumothorax
- Tamponade
- Toxic/therapeutic disorders
- Thromboembolism
Check: electrode positions and contact
Attempt/verify: IV/IO access
Give: adrenaline (epinephrine) every 3–5 min.
Consider: amiodarone, atropine, magnesium

GP Notes:

Estimating the weight of a child for drug/fluid doses:

- May not be necessary – use a recent weight from the parent-held child record if available.
- Otherwise for children >1y., weight (in kg) ≈ 2x (age + 4).

Figure 1.6 is reproduced with permission from the Resuscitation Guidelines (2005)
🖳 www.resus.org.uk

Recovery position

When circulation and breathing have been restored, it is important to:
- Maintain a good airway
- Ensure the tongue does not cause obstruction
- Minimize the risk of inhalation of gastric contents.

For this reason the victim should be placed in the recovery position. This allows the tongue to fall forward, keeping the airway clear.

Putting a patient in the recovery position: See Figure 1.7
- Remove the patient's glasses.
- Kneel beside the patient and make sure that both legs are straight (A).
- Place the arm nearest to you out at right angles to the body, elbow bent with the hand palm uppermost (A).
- Bring the far arm across the chest, and hold the back of the hand against the patient's cheek nearest to you (B).
- With your other hand, grasp the far leg just above the knee and pull it up, keeping the foot on the ground (B).
- Keeping the patient's hand pressed against his cheek, pull on the leg to roll the patient towards you onto his side (C).
- Adjust the upper leg so that both the hip and knee are bent at right angles (D).
- Tilt the head back to make sure the airway remains open (D).
- Adjust the hand under the cheek, if necessary, to keep the head tilted (D).
- Check breathing regularly.

⚠ Monitor the peripheral circulation of the lower arm. If the patient has to be kept in the recovery position for >30min., turn the patient onto the opposite side.

The unconscious child:
- The child should be in as near a true lateral position as possible with his mouth dependent to allow free drainage of fluid.
- The position should be stable. In an infant this may require the support of a small pillow or rolled-up blanket placed behind the infant's back to maintain the position.

Cervical spine injury:
- If spinal cord injury is suspected (for example if the victim has sustained a fall, been struck on the head or neck, or has been rescued after diving into shallow water), take particular care during handling and resuscitation to maintain alignment of the head, neck and chest in the neutral position.
- A spinal board and/or cervical collar should be used if available.

Figure 1.7 Recovery position

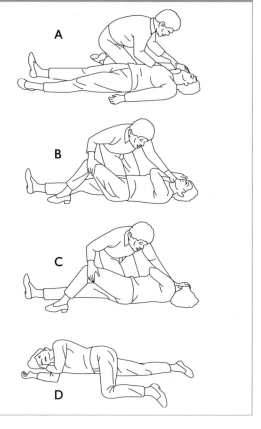

Chapter 2

Assessing patients with cardiac and vascular problems in primary care

21

Cardiac and vascular assessment

When assessing a patient with suspected cardiac or vascular problems in primary care, the objectives are to:

- Establish a constructive relationship with the patient to enable patient and doctor to communicate effectively, and serve as the basis for any subsequent therapeutic relationship.
- Determine whether the patient has a problem and, if so, what that is.
- Find out (where possible) what caused that problem.
- Assess the patient's emotions and attitudes towards the problem.
- Establish how it might be treated.

History: Use open questions at the start, becoming directive when necessary – clarify, reflect, facilitate, listen. Ask *about*:

Presenting complaint: Chronological account, past history of similar symptoms (Figure 2.1).

Chest pain and palpitations: 📖 p.38   *Dyspnoea:* 📖 p.40

Past medical history
- Previous cardiac disease e.g. MI/angina, arrhythmia, congenital heart disease, valve disease or valve replacement, heart transplant
- Risk factors for cardiovascular disease e.g. ↑ BP, hypercholesterolaemia, DM, ankylosing spondylitis, acromegaly
- Previous cerebrovascular disease e.g. stroke, amaurosis fugax
- Previous venous disease e.g. DVT, varicose veins
- Past treatments e.g. surgery, current medication, medications previously tried

Family history
- Cardiovascular problems e.g. cardiomyopathy, premature stroke or atherosclerotic heart disease
- Risk factors for cardiovascular disease e.g. ↑ BP, hypercholesterolaemia
- Venous disease e.g. DVT, varicose veins, thrombophilia

Social history: Smoking history. Alcohol consumption. Employed? Does the problem affect the job? Housing, social support etc.

Attitudes and beliefs: How does the patient see the problem? What does s/he think is wrong? How does s/he think other people view the situation? What does s/he want you to do about it?

Examination: Figure 2.1

Investigation: Figure 2.1

Action
- Summarize the history back to the patient and give an opportunity for the patient to fill in any gaps.
- Draw up a problem list and outline a management plan with the patient. Further investigations and interventions are guided by the findings on history and examination – so a good history and examination is essential.
- Set a review date.

Figure 2.1 Cardiac and vascular assessment

ASK

Chronological history of symptoms:

Venous disease
Pain/swelling of leg?
Fever?
Varicose veins?
Varicose eczema?
Otherskin changes?
Leg ulcer?
Chest pain/breathlessness?

Cardiac disease
Chest pain?
Dysponoea?
Ankle swelling?
Palpitaitons?
Fatigue?
Dizziness or blackouts?

Peripheral arterial disease
Intermittent claudication?
Rest pain?

Cerebrovascular disease
Neurological symptoms?
Visual symptoms?
Dizziness or blackouts?

Past meical history, family and social history

EXAMINE

Tailor examination to confirm/refute suspected diagnosis and
identify risk factors. Consider:
– General examination – hands, eyes, peripheral oedema,
  scars ± temperature (if any suggestion of infection) – p.24
– Check BP – p.28
– Examine neck – carotid pulse, bruits, JVP – p.30
– Examine chest – apex beat, heart sounds, murmurs/thrills, basal
  crepitaions – p.32
– Check abdomen for hepatomegaly and AAA (p.36)_
– Check peripheral pulses – p.36–7
– Check neurology if history of visual/neurological deficit
– Examine legs for DVT (p.146) and/or varicose veins (p.140)

INVESTIGATE

Consider:
ECG/ambulatory ECG/exercise ECG – p.52
Echo – p..54
Ankle brachial pressure index (ABPI) – p.37
Carotid dopplers/dopplers of other arteries – p.54
Referral for specialist investigation

General examination

General inspection: Watch the patient throughout the consultation:
- How did he walk into the room? Was he breathless on exertion?
- Does the patient have a syndrome associated with cardiac abnormalities e.g. Turner's syndrome, Down's syndrome, Marfan's syndrome?
- Does the patient have another condition associated with heart disease e.g. obesity, cachexia (associated with chronic heart failure), ankylosing spondylitis?
- Does the patient appear breathless whilst talking?
- How does he get onto the examination couch?
- Is he in obvious discomfort or distress?
- Are there any scars indicative of previous cardiac or vascular surgery?

Jaundice: In the context of suspected heart disease may be due to hepatic engorgement due to heart failure (often accompanied by hepatomegaly) or haemolysis due to prosthetic heart valves.

Cyanosis: Dusky blue skin.
Central cyanosis: Cyanosis of mucous membranes e.g. mouth. *Causes:*
- Lung disease resulting in inadequate oxygen transfer (e.g. COPD, PE, pleural effusion, severe chest infection)
- Shunting from pulmonary to systemic circulation (e.g. Fallot's tetralogy, PDA, transposition of the great arteries)
- Inadequate oxygen uptake (e.g. met- or sulf-haemoglobinaemia).

Peripheral cyanosis: e.g. cyanosis of fingers. *Causes:* as for central cyanosis plus:
- Physiological (cold, hypovolaemia)
- Local arterial disease (e.g. Raynaud's syndrome).

❶ Feet can be a dusky blue colour due to venous disease too. When this occurs without central cyanosis it does not imply abnormal oxygen saturation.

Mitral facies: Dusky bluish red flushing of the cheeks (a form of peripheral cyanosis) associated with a low cardiac output.

Clubbing: Loss of the angle between nail fold and plate, bulbous finger tip and the nail fold feels boggy (Figure 2.2). *Causes:*
- *Cardiac:* SBE; congenital cyanotic heart disease
- *Respiratory:* bronchial carcinoma (not small cell); chronic infection; fibrosing alveolitis; asbestosis
- *Other:* inflammatory bowel disease (Crohn's > UC); thyrotoxicosis; biliary cirrhosis; congenital; A-V malformation

Signs of infective endocarditis
- *Infective:* fever, weight ↓, clubbing, splenomegaly, anaemia.
- *Cardiac:* murmurs (particularly new murmurs) ± heart failure
- *Embolic:* neurologic deficit due to stroke
- *Vasculitic:* Figure 2.3 – microscopic haematuria, splinter haemorrhages, conjunctival haemorrhages, Roth's spots (retinal vasculitis), Osler's nodes (painful lesions on finger pulps), Janeway's lesions (palmar macules)

Figure 2.2 Clubbed finger nail

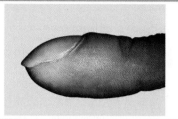

Figure 2.3 Vasculitic signs of infective endocarditis

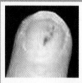

(a) Splinter haemorrhages: normally seen under the fingernails. Linear and red for the first 2–3d. and brownish thereafter

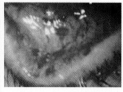

(b) Conjunctival petechiae

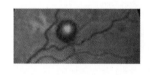

(c) Roth's spot: white retinal lesion with surrounding haemorrhage

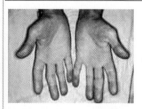

(d) Osler's nodes: tender, subcutaneous nodules usually in the finger pulps or thenar eminence

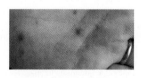

(e) Janeway's lesions: non-tender, erythematous, haemorrhagic or pustular lesions, often on palms or soles

Figure 2.2 is reproduced with permission from dermnet.com
Figure 2.3 is reproduced with permission from Cambridge University School of Clinical Pharmacy

Peripheral oedema: Swelling of the ankles/legs (or sacrum if bed bound) occurs when the rate of capillary filtration > rate drainage.
- Increased capillary filtration occurs due to ↑ venous pressure, hypoalbuminaemia or local inflammation.
- Decreased drainage occurs due to lymphatic obstruction.

Consider whether the swelling is acute or chronic, symmetrical or asymmetrical, localised or generalised. Ask about associated symptoms e.g. breathlessness. Treat according to cause:

Acute
- DVT
- Superficial thrombophlebitis
- Cellulitis
- Joint effusion/haemarthrosis
- Haematoma
- Baker's cyst
- Arthritis
- Fracture
- Acute arterial ischaemia
- Dermatitis

Chronic
- Gravitational oedema e.g due to immobility – common in the elderly – advise elevation of feet above waist level, support stockings (ideally apply stockings before getting out of bed), avoid standing still. Diuretics are not a long-term solution
- Heart failure
- Hypoproteinaemia e.g. nephrotic syndrome
- Idiopathic oedema
- Reflex sympathetic dystrophy
- Lymphoedema – infection, tumour, trauma
- Post-thrombotic syndrome
- Chronic venous insufficiency/venous obstruction
- Lipodermatosclerosis
- Congenital vascular abnormalities

Signs of hypercholesterolaemia

Corneal arcus: Whitish opaque line surrounding the margin of the cornea, separated from it by an area of clear cornea (Figure 2.4). Rarely congenital – more commonly occurs bilaterally in patients >50y. (arcus senilis). Sometimes associated with ↑ blood lipids – particularly familial hypercholesterolaemias. Check lipids. If lipids are normal, no treatment is needed.

Xanthomata: Localized collections of lipid-laden cells. Appear as yellowish-coloured lumps. Often caused by ↑ lipids. Commonly seen on the eyelids (xanthelasma – Figure 2.5), on the skin, or in tendons (appear as mobile nodules in the tendon).

Figure 2.4 Corneal arcus

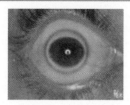

Figure 2.5 Xanthelasma: small, pale lesions in superficial skin layers

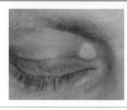

gures 2.4 and 2.5 are reproduced with permission from Southampton University Hospitals ust.

Blood pressure measurement

Taking blood pressure

- Regularly maintain and calibrate your sphygmomanometer.
- Use a cuff of correct width:
  - *Most adults* – 12 x 26cm bladder size
  - *Large adults (arm circumference >33cm)* – 12 x 40cm bladder size
  - *Thin adults and children with arm circumference ≤ 26cm* –
    10 x 18cm bladder size.
- Seat the patient with arm at the level of the heart.
- In patients with symptoms of postural hypotension (falls or dizziness measure BP when standing. If drop in systolic BP of >20mmHg consider specialist referral.
- Measure BP to nearest 2mmHg.
- Measure diastolic pressure when heart sounds completely disappear (K_5). (Only use the pressure at which they suddenly muffle (K_4) wher K_5 cannot be determined.)
- BP varies throughout the day and can ↑ as a response to having BP checked ('white-coat phenomenon' – prevalence 10%). Take ≥2 measurements on 2 occasions before classifying a patient as hypertensive.
- BP measurements should normally be made at monthly intervals, but should be done more frequently in severe hypertension.
- If BP is very variable, consider ambulatory BP monitoring (gives average BP over 24h.) or intermittent home BP monitoring.

Home monitoring and ambulatory BP monitoring: Both ma have advantages in eliminating variation between readings (by taking th average), in decreasing white-coat hypertension, and in reduce observer bias. Finger and wrist devices are not recommended. Elec tronic devices for patient use loaned from GP premises are popular bu require regular calibration and maintenance and not all patients adher to instructions for use.

Table 2.1 Threshold values for treatment for ambulatory BP monitoring	
	Abnormal
Daytime	>140/90
Night-time	>125/75
24 hours	>135/85

The threshold for treatment for home monitoring is usually taken a 135/85.

The British Hypertension Society recommend downward adjustment c clinic readings by 12/7mmHg, in order to make a valid comparison wit home monitoring reading.

❗ NICE does not recommend the routine use of ambulatory or hom BP monitoring methods at present due to lack of research evidence.

Hypertension: 📖 p.168

Hypotension: Suggests fluid loss or heart pump failure.

Postural hypotension: BP drops on moving from supine or sitting position to standing position. Confirm diagnosis by checking BP lying and then standing. Standing usually causes a slight ↓ in the systolic BP (<20mmHg) and a slight ↑ in the diastolic BP (<10mmHg). In postural hypotension there is usually a marked ↓ in both systolic and diastolic BP.

Review medication: Stop any non-essential medication contributing to symptoms e.g. night sedation, unnecessary diuretics.

Optimize treatment of intercurrent heart disease, Parkinson's disease or DM.

Advice: Patients should take care when standing, especially if getting up from their beds or out of a hot bath/shower, and after meals.

Cardiogenic shock: Due to heart pump failure e.g. MI, arrythmia, tamponade. *Signs:*

Hypotension – systolic BP <80–90mmHg

Pulse rate may be normal, ↑ or ↓

Severe breathlessness ± cyanosis

Pallor and sweating

⚠ **Acute management of cardiogenic shock**

- Sit the patient up if possible.
- Call for ambulance assistance.
- Treat any underlying cause found e.g. atropine for bradycardia; diamorphine, frusemide and GTN spray for acute LVF.
- Gain IV access if possible.
- If available give 100% oxygen (unless COPD when give 24%).

29

GMS contract		
Records 11	BP of patients aged ≥45y. is recorded in the preceding 5y. for ≥65% of patients	10 points
Records 17	BP of patients aged ≥45y. is recorded in the preceding 5y. for ≥80% of patients	5 points
Management 7	The practice has systems in place to ensure regular and appropriate inspection, calibration, maintenance and replacement of equipment* including: • A defined responsible person • Clear recording • Systematic pre-planned schedules • Reporting of faults	3 points

* This includes BP machines.

Neck signs

Ask the patient to lie supine with head/neck at 45° to the horizontal.

Carotid pulse: When assessing the carotid pulse, consider:

Rate
- *Tachycardia:* >100bpm – 🕮 p.88
- *Bradycardia:* <60bpm – 🕮 p.96

Rhythm
- *Irregularly irregular:* AF, multiple ectopics
- *Regularly irregular:* 2nd degree heart block

Character and volume: Always assess with a central pulse e.g. carotid or femoral.
- *Small volume:* Shock, pericardial tamponade, aortic stenosis (slow-rising)
- *Large volume:* Hyperdynamic circulation (e.g. pregnancy), aortic incompetence (water-hammer, collapsing pulse), PDA.
- *Pulsus paradoxus:* Pulse weakens in inspiration by >10mmHg – asthma, cardiac tamponade, pericarditis

Carotid bruits: May signify stenosis (>30%) often near the origin of internal carotid. Heard best behind the angle of the jaw. Usual cause is atheroma.

Jugular venous pressure: Observe internal jugular vein at 45° with head turned slightly to the left. Vertical height is measured in relation to the sternal angle. Raised if >4cm.

Causes of ↑ JVP
- Fluid overload
- Right heart failure and CCF
- SVC obstruction (non-pulsatile)
- Tricuspid or pulmonary valve disease
- Pulmonary hypertension
- Arrythmia – AF or atrial flutter, complete heart block
- ↑ intrathoracic pressure e.g. pneumothorax, PE, emphysema

Kussmaul's sign: The JVP usually drops on inspiration along with intrathoracic pressure. The reverse pattern is called Kussmaul's sign. Caused by raised intrathoracic pressure or constrictive pericarditis.

Wave patterns: Figure 2.6
- *A wave:* Due to right atrial systole; coincides with the 1st heart sound; precedes the carotid pulse.
- *C wave:* Due to transmission of right ventricular pressure before the tricuspid valve closes. Rarely visible.
- *X descent:* Due to relaxation of the right atrium.
- *V wave:* Due to venous blood filling the right atrium whilst the tricuspid valve is closed as the ventricles contract. Occurs at the same time as the carotid pulse.
- *Y descent:* Due to opening of the tricuspid valve when the ventricles relax.

Abnormal wave patterns: Table 2.2

GP Notes: Finding the carotid pulse

- Tilt the head towards the side being examined to relax the sternomastoid muscle.
- Palpate lateral to the upper trachea/lower larynx (Adam's apple) and medial to the sternomastoid.
- Never palpate both carotid arteries simultaneously.

Figure 2.6 Jugular venous pressure wave

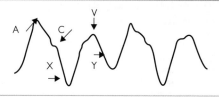

Table 2.2 Abnormal JVP wave patterns and their causes

Condition	Abnormal wave pattern
Tricuspid regurgitation	Large systolic wave which replaces the C and V wave with steep Y descent
Tricuspid stenosis	Large A wave; small V wave, slow Y descent
Complete heart block, VT or other causes of atrioventricular dissociation	Cannon waves: very large A waves which occur when the right atrium contracts against a closed tricuspid valve
AF	Absent A wave, C wave normal
Constrictive pericarditis	Kussmaul's sign, steep Y descent

Examination of the chest

Apex beat
- The normal position of the apex beat of the heart is the 5th intercostal space, in (or just medial to) the midclavicular line.
- Infants and children have apex beats which are superior and more lateral to those of adults.
- Apex beat may not be palpable if the patient is obese, has hyperexpanded lungs (e.g. COPD) or a pericardial effusion.
- The apex beat is moved sideways or inferiorly if the heart is enlarged (e.g. CCF) or displaced (e.g. pneumothorax).

Parasternal heave: Detect by placing the heel of the hand over the left parasternal region. When a heave is present, the heel of the hand is lifted off the chest wall with each heartbeat. *Causes:* Usually due to right ventricular enlargement – rarely due to left atrial enlargement.

Crackles in the chest: Produced by air flow moving secretions from airways or lung tissue.
- *Fine crackles:* Consider pulmonary oedema (early inspiratory – usually best heard at the lung bases at the back); early pneumonia; fibrosing alveolitis (late inspiratory).
- *Coarse crackles:* Consider TB; resolving pneumonia; bronchiectasis; lung abscess.

Heart sounds
Ausculation: Auscultation areas – Figure 2.7
- *Low and medium frequency sounds* (e.g. 3rd and 4th heart sounds) are more easily heard with the bell applied lightly to the skin.
- *High frequency sounds* (e.g. 1st and 2nd heart sounds and opening snaps) are more easily heard with a diaphragm.

Interpretation of heart sounds: Table 2.4 (📖 p.35).

Heart murmurs

⚠ Red flag symptoms	
• Cyanosis	• Collapse
• Breathlessness	• Weight loss (or failure to thrive
• Lethargy and tiredness	in children)

Due to abnormalities of flow within the heart and great vessels. Very common. Often incidental finding. Described by:
- *Location* – where heard loudest
- *Quality* e.g. blowing, harsh
- *Intensity* – graded out of 6, 1 being virtually undetectable and 6 being heard by an observer without a stethoscope (grades 4–6 are usually palpable as well as audible)
- *Timing* – systolic or diastolic, *and*
- *Radiation* – does the murmur spread elsewhere e.g. to axilla, carotids.

Always refer for echocardiographic confirmation.

Differential diagnosis: Table 2.3

Figure 2.7 Auscultation areas

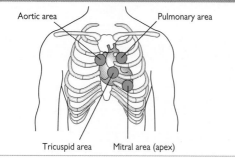

Aortic area   Pulmonary area

Tricuspid area   Mitral area (apex)

Table 2.3 Differential diagnosis of heart murmurs

Type of murmur	Description	Causes
Ejection systolic murmur	↑ to reach a peak midway between the heart sounds.	• Flow murmurs e.g children, pregnancy, with fever, during/after exercise • Aortic stenosis or sclerosis (📖 p.114) • Pulmonary stenosis (📖 p.116) • HOCM (📖 p.106)
Pan-systolic murmur	Uniform intensity between the 2 heart sounds. Merges with 2nd heart sound.	• Mitral valve regurgitation or prolapse (📖 p.112) • Tricuspid regurgitation (📖 p.116) • VSD (📖 p.120) • ASD (📖 p.118)
Early diastolic murmur	Occurs just after the 2nd heart sound. High pitched and easily missed.	• Aortic regurgitation (📖 p.116) • Pulmonary regurgitation (📖 p.116) • Tricuspid stenosis (mitral stenosis co-exists)
Mid-diastolic murmur	Midway between 2nd heart sound of 1 beat and 1st of the next. Rumbling and low pitched.	• Mitral stenosis (📖 p.114) • Aortic regurgitation. (Austin Flint murmur – 📖 p.116)

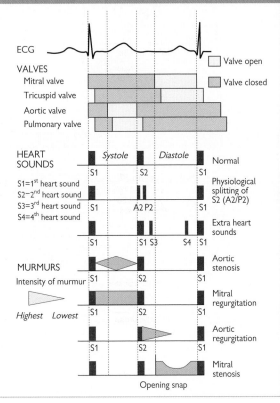

Figure 2.8 Relationship of heart sounds and murmurs to the ECG and valve function

Table 2.4 Heart sounds, abnormalities and their causes

Heart sound		Causes
1st heart sound Heard loudest at the apex. Caused by closing of the mitral and tricuspid valves.	Soft	Mitral regurgitation, low BP, rheumatic carditis, severe heart failure, LBBB
	Loud	AF, tachycardia, atrial premature beat, mitral stenosis
	Variable intensity	Varying duration of diastole, complete AV block
	Split	RBBB, paced beat from the left ventricle, left ventricular ectopics, ASD, Ebstein's anomaly, tricuspid stenosis
2nd heart sound Caused by closure of the aortic (A2) and pulmonary (P2) valves. A2 and P2 split on inspiration so that P2 is heard after A2.	Soft	• A2 – calcification of the aortic valve, dilatation of the aortic root • P2 – pulmonary stenosis
	Loud	• A2 – ↑BP, thin patients • P2 – pulmonary hypertension, ASD
	Wide splitting	May be the result of early A2 or delayed P2. • Early A2 – mitral regurgitation, VSD • Delayed P2 – RBBB, pulmonary stenosis, ASD, right ventricular failure
	Reversed splitting	A2 is delayed. P2 occurs before A2 so the split between the sounds ↓ on inspiration. Delayed A2 – LBBB, systolic hypertension, HOCM, severe aortic stenosis, PDA, left heart failure
	Single	Calcification of the aortic valve, pulmonary stenosis, Fallot's tetralogy, Ebstein's anomaly, pericardial effusion, large VSD, obesity, emphysema
Clicks and snaps	Early systolic	Caused by opening of the aortic or pulmonary valves • Aortic – aortic stenosis, bicuspid valve • Pulmonary – pulmonary stenosis, pulmonary hypertension
	Mid/late systolic	Mitral valve prolapse
	Diastolic	Caused by opening of the mitral or tricuspid valves. Silent in the healthy heart. • Mitral – mitral stenosis, rapid mitral flow e.g. PDA, VSD, severe mitral regurgitation • Tricuspid (rare) – rheumatic stenosis, ASD
3rd heart sound Heard in diastole after the 2nd heart sound.	Right ventricle	Loudest at lower left sternal edge. Never normal. Causes – right heart failure, tricuspid regurgitation, ASD, constrictive pericarditis
	Left ventricle	Loudest at the apex when inclined to the left. Can be normal in children and pregnancy. Other causes: LVF, mitral regurgitation, anterior MI
4th heart sound Heard in late diastole.		Maximal at the apex or lower left sternal edge. Never normal. Causes: ventricular hypertrophy or fibrosis and HOCM

Examination of the arterial vascular system

The main conditions affecting the abdominal and peripheral arteries are:
- Aneurysms (📖 p.130)
- Atherosclerosis resulting in ischaemia of the legs and intermittent claudication, atrophic changes and/or rest pain
- Embolization resulting in acute ischaemia of the limbs.

General scheme
- Look at the limbs – are there any signs of ischaemia? Are the extremities warm or cold? What colour are they?
- Examine the abdomen looking for a pulsatile mass which might suggest abdominal aortic aneurysm. Auscultation may reveal a bruit.
- Check the peripheral pulses.

⚠ Tenderness on palpation of an abdominal aortic aneurysm suggests need for urgent operative repair.

Peripheral pulses
Location: Table 2.5

Examination: Check whether each pulse is present. If present check:
- Rate
- Rhythm
- Amplitude
- Compare pulses in the 2 legs/2 arms.

Check for radiofemoral delay – palpate radial and femoral pulses simultaneously – delay suggests coarctation of the aorta.

Check for bruits over the femoral and/or carotid pulses – indicate disturbed blood flow – usually secondary to narrowing due to atherosclerosis.

⚠ Character and waveform of the pulse should *only* be assessed using the femoral or carotid pulse (📖 p.30).

Signs of ischaemia
Acute ischaemia: Acutely pale, cold and pulseless limb – 📖 p.135 Refer immediately – keep the limb cool in the interim.

Chronic ischaemic changes:
- Atrophic skin changes – pallor, cool to the touch, hairless, shiny
- On lowering the leg turns a dusky blue–red colour; on elevation – pallor and venous guttering
- Ulceration – check under the heel and between the toes
- Swelling suggests the patient is sleeping in a chair to avoid rest pain or, rarely, pain from deep infection
- Absent foot pulses – if pulses are present consider alternative diagnosis
- Ankle-brachial pressure index <0.95 (see opposite)

Table 2.5 Location of the limb pulses

Pulse	Location
Brachial	~2cm medial to the central point of the antecubital fossa over the elbow skin crease
Radial	~½ –1cm on the radial (lateral) side of the flexor carpi radialis tendon at the wrist
Femoral	Below inguinal ligament; $^1/_3$ of the way up from pubic tubercle
Popliteal	With knee flexed at right angles, palpate deep in the midline
Posterior tibial	1cm behind medial malleolus
Dorsalis pedis	Variable – on the dorsum of the foot just lateral to the tendons to the big toe. ⓘ Many healthy people have only 1 foot pulse

GP Notes: Checking the ankle–brachial pressure index (ABPI)

- Check BP in one arm (📖 p.28). The systolic measurement is the brachial pressure (B).
- Then inflate a BP cuff around the lower calf just above the ankle.
- Using a Doppler ultrasound probe, record the maximum cuff pressure at which the probe can still record a pulse (ankle pressure – A).
- Calculate the ankle–brachial pressure index by dividing the ankle pressure by the brachial pressure i.e. ABPI = A ÷ B.

Interpretation of ABPI results

- ABPI <0.95 – ischaemia
- ABPI <0.5 – critical ischaemia

ⓘ Arterial calcification (e.g. due to DM) can result in falsely elevated ankle pressure readings.

Chest pain and palpitations

Chest pain: Common symptom.

⚠ Always think – could this be an MI, PE, dissecting aneurysm or pericarditis?

On receiving the call for assistance: Ask:
- Nature and location of the pain
- Duration of the pain
- Other associated symptoms – sweating, nausea, shortness of breath, palpitations
- Past medical history (particularly heart disease, high cholesterol)
- Family history (particularly heart disease)
- Smoker?

Action
- Consider differential diagnosis (Table 2.6).
- If MI is suspected, call for ambulance assistance before (or instead of) visiting.
- Otherwise visit (or arrange surgery appointment), assess and treat according to cause.

Further assessment
History: Ask about:
- Site and nature of pain
- Duration
- Associated symptoms (e.g. breathlessness, nausea)
- Provoking and relieving factors
- PMH, FH (e.g. heart disease), drug history, smoking history

Examination
- Check BP in both arms
- General appearance – distress, sweating, pallor
- JVP
- Carotid pulse
- Apex beat
- Heart sounds
- Lung fields
- Local tenderness
- Pain on movement of chest
- Skin rashes
- Swelling or tenderness of legs (?DVT)

Investigations: ECG and CXR may be helpful.

Palpitations: The uncomfortable awareness of heartbeat. Can be physiological (e.g. after exercise, at times of stress) or signify arrhythmia. Can cause a feeling of faintness or even collapse (e.g. Stokes-Adams attack, due to AV block). Ask the patient to tap out the rhythm.
- *Bradycardia:* 📖 p.96
- *Occasional missed beat:* suggests ventricular ectopics – 📖 p.90
- *Tachycardia:* 📖 p.88

Table 2.6 Causes of acute chest pain

Diagnosis	Features
MI	Band-like chest pain around the chest or central chest pressure/dull ache ± radiation to shoulders, arms (L>R), neck and/or jaw. Often associated with nausea, sweating and/or shortness of breath.
Unstable angina	As for MI.
Pericarditis	Sharp, constant sternal pain relieved by sitting forwards. May radiate to left shoulder ± arm or into the abdomen. Worse lying on the left side and on inspiration, swallowing and coughing.
Dissecting thoracic aneurysm	Typically presents with sudden tearing chest pain radiating to the back. Consider in any patient with chest pain (especially if radiates through to the back) and ↓BP.
PE	Acute dyspnoea, sharp chest pain (worse on inspiration), haemoptysis and/or syncope. Tachycardic and mild pyrexia.
Pleurisy	Sharp, localized chest pain, worse on inspiration. May be associated with symptoms and signs of a chest infection.
Pneumothorax	Sudden onset of pleuritic chest pain or ↑ breathlessness ± pallor and tachycardia.
Oesophageal spasm, oesophagitis	Central chest pain. May be associated with acid reflux (though not always). May be described as burning but often indistinguishable from cardiac pain. May respond to antacids.
Musculoskeletal pain	Localized pain – worse on movement. May be a history of injury or coughing.
Shingles	Intense, often sharp, unilateral pain. Responds poorly to analgesia. May be present several days before rash appears.
Costochondritis	Inflammation of the costochondral junctions – tenderness over the costochondral junction and pain in the affected area on springing the chest wall.
Bornholm's disease	Unilateral chest and/or abdominal pain, rhinitis. Coxsackie virus infection. Treat with simple analgesia.
Idiopathic chest pain	No cause apparent. Common. Affects young people > elderly people. ♀>♂

GP Notes:

⚠ If a patient is acutely unwell with chest pain and the cause is not clear, err on the side of caution and admit for further assessment.

Dyspnoea

Dyspnoea: Sensation of shortness of breath. Speed of onset helps diagnosis (Table 2.7). Try to quantify exercise tolerance (e.g. dressing, distance walked, climbing stairs).

Acute breathlessness: Attend as soon as possible after receiving the call for help. If there is likely to be any delay, call for emergency ambulance assistance.

On arrival

- Be calm and reassuring. Breathlessness is frightening and panic only adds to the sensation of being breathless.
- Direct history and examination to find the cause as quickly as possible (Table 2.7). Treat according to the cause.
- If no cause can be found – don't delay – admit to hospital as an acute medical emergency.

Exertional dyspnoea: Breathlessness with exercise. Causes are the same as dyspnoea generally. The New York Heart Association classifies 4 grades of severity:

- *Normal*
- *Moderate:* Walking on the level causes breathlessness.
- *Severe:* Has to stop due to breathlessness when walking on the flat. All but the lightest housework is impossible.
- *Gross:* Slightest effort → severe breathlessness. The patient is almost bed/chair bound.

Orthopnoea: Dyspnoea on lying flat and relieved by sitting up. Associated with left heart dysfunction e.g. LVF.

Paroxysmal nocturnal dyspnoea: Acute form of dyspnoea that causes the patient to awake from sleep. The patient is forced to sit upright or stand out of bed for relief. Associated with pulmonary oedema.

Combined chest pain and dyspnoea: *Consider:*

- MI
- Pericarditis
- Dissecting aneurysm
- PE
- Oesophageal pain
- Musculoskeletal pain
- Chest infection
- Pulmonary malignancy e.g. mesothelioma, lung cancer

Table 2.7 Causes of dyspnoea

Cause	Acute	Subacute	Chronic
Cardiac disease	Acute LVF Arrhythmia Air hunger due to shock e.g. 2° to MI, dissecting thoracic aneurysm Pericarditis	Arrhythmia SBE	CCF Mitral stenosis Aortic stenosis Congenital heart disease
Lung disease	Pneumothorax Acute asthma attack PE Acute pneumonitis e.g. due to inhaling toxic gas	Asthma Infective Exacerbation of COPD Pleural effusion Pneumonia	COPD Cystic fibrosis Fibrosing alveolitis Occupational lung diseases Mesothelioma Lung cancer
Other	Hyperventilation Foreign body inhalation Guillain-Barré syndrome Altitude sickness Ketoacidosis Polio Musculoskeletal chest pain Oesophageal pain	Aspirin poisoning Myaesthenia gravis Thyrotoxicosis	Kyphoscoliosis Anaemia MND MS

The electrocardiogram (ECG)

ECGs are graphic recordings of electric potentials generated by the heart. They provide diagnostic information for a variety of cardiac and systemic diseases (e.g. renal failure, thyroid disease).

Positioning of leads for a standard 12-lead ECG

Limb leads: Locate on a boney area to minimize skeletal muscle interference.
- Right arm – red lead
- Left arm – yellow lead
- Left leg – green lead
- Right leg – black lead

Information from limb electrodes is combined to produce the 6 limb leads (I, II, III, aVR, aVL, and aVF – Figure 2.9), which view the heart in a vertical plane.

Chest leads: The 6 chest leads (V1 to V6) view the heart in a horizontal plane – Figure 2.10.
- V1 – 4th intercostal space, right sternal border
- V2 – 4th intercostal space, left sternal border
- V3 – Midway between V2 and V4
- V4 – 5th intercostal space, mid clavicular line
- V5 – Anterior axillary line, horizontal to V4
- V6 – Mid axillary line, horizontal to V4 and V5

ⓘ V4, 5 and 6 do **not** follow the 5th intercostal space.

Anatomical relations of leads: In a standard 12-lead ECG:
- II, III, and aVF – inferior surface of the heart
- V1–V4 – anterior surface
- I, aVL, V5, and V6 – lateral surface
- V1 and aVR – right atrium and cavity of left ventricle

Speed and calibration

Speed: The ECG is recorded onto standard paper travelling at a rate of 25mm/s. The paper is divided into large squares, each measuring 5mm wide and equivalent to 0.2s. Each large square is 5 small squares in width, and each small square is 1mm wide and equivalent to 0.04s.

Calibration: Electrical activity detected by the ECG machine is measured in millivolts (mV). Machines are calibrated so that a signal with amplitude of 1mV moves the recording stylus 1cm vertically – therefore 0.1mV = 1mm = 1 small square.

Interpreting ECGs: 📖 p.44

Common ECG changes and their causes: 📖 pp.46–51

Further information

Hampton *The ECG made easy* (2003) Churchill Livingstone ISBN: 0443072523

Morris et al. *ABC of clinical electrocardiography* (2002) BMJ Books ISBN: 0727915363

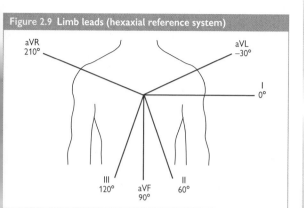

Figure 2.9 Limb leads (hexaxial reference system)

aVR 210°
aVL −30°
I 0°
III 120°
aVF 90°
II 60°

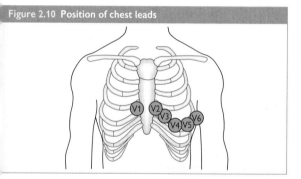

Figure 2.10 Position of chest leads

GMS contract		
Management 7	The practice has systems in place to ensure regular and appropriate inspection, calibration, maintenance and replacement of equipment including: • A defined responsible person • Clear recording • Systematic pre-planned schedules • Reporting of faults	3 points

Figure 2.10 is reproduced from Morris F, Edhouse J, Brady W, and Camm J, (2002), The *ABC of Clinical Electrocardiography*, with permission from Blackwell BMJ Books.

Interpreting ECGs: Many surgeries now have ECG machines that interpret themselves and print out their findings. Analysis is easier but it is still important to be able to understand significance of abnormalities and check computer analysis in the clinical context. Many mistakes in ECG interpretation are errors of omission so a systematic approach is best.

Check:

1. **Standardization** (calibration – Figure 2.11) and **technical features** (including lead placement and artifacts)

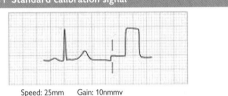

Figure 2.11 **Standard calibration signal**

Speed: 25mm   Gain: 10nmmv

2. **Heart rate** – usual speed (25mm/s). Each big square represents 0.2s. (small square – 0.04s.). Rate = 300 ÷ R–R interval in large squares
3. **Rhythm** – regular/irregular
4. **PR interval** – normal if <0.2s.
5. **QRS interval** – abnormal if >0.12s.
6. **QT interval** – varies with rate. At 60bpm normal if 0.35–0.43s.
7. **P waves** – present or absent, shape
8. **QRS voltages** – height of complexes – see Figure 2.13, 📖 p.45
9. **Mean QRS electrical axis** – sum of all ventricular forces during ventricular depolarization. Normal axis: −30° to +120°. If more −ve than −30° = left axis deviation. If more +ve than +120° = right axis deviation
10. **Pre-cordial R-wave progression** – Figure 2.12

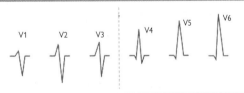

Figure 2.12 **Pre-cordial R-wave progression**

V1   V2   V3   V4   V5   V6

11. **Abnormal Q waves** – abnormal if >25% of the succeeding R wave and/or >0.04s. wide
11. **ST segments** – elevation/depression, shape
12. **T waves** – height, inversion, shape
13. **U waves** – small, rounded deflection (≤1mm), follows T wave and usually has the same polarity

Figures 2.11 and 2.12 are reproduced from Morris F, Edhouse J, Brady W, and Camm J, (2002) The *ABC of Clinical Electrocardiography*, with permission from Blackwell BMJ Books.

Figure 2.13 The PQRST complex

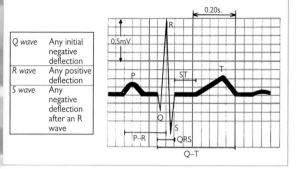

Q wave	Any initial negative deflection
R wave	Any positive deflection
S wave	Any negative deflection after an R wave

GP Notes: Calculating the cardiac axis

Rule of thumb 1: If the majority of the QRS complex is above the baseline (+ve) in leads I and II, the axis is normal.

Rule of thumb 2: The axis lies at 90° to a QRS complex where the height above the baseline = height below the baseline (equiphasic lead).

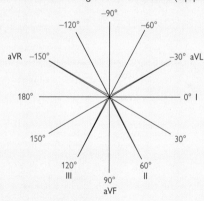

With reference to the diagram – inspect the QRS complexes in the leads adjacent to the equiphasic lead:

- If the lead to the left side is positive, then the axis is at 90° to the equiphasic lead towards the left.
- If the lead to the right side is positive, then the axis is 90° to the equiphasic lead towards the right.

Table 2.8 Common ECG abnormalities and their causes

ECG abnormality		Figure	Possible causes
Tachycardia	Rate >100bpm	2.14 (a)	Physiological, AF, atrial flutter, SVT, VT.
Bradycardia	Rate <60bpm	2.14 (b)	Physiological, drugs (e.g. β-blockers, digoxin), heart block (see 📖 p.96), sick sinus syndrome
Irregular	Assess whether any pattern or not	2.14 (c)	AF (no pattern), sick sinus syndrome (no pattern), ventricular ectopics (normally no pattern), heart block (pattern)
P–R interval	Short P–R interval	2.15 (a)	Nodal rhythm, Wolf-Parkinson-White syndrome (📖 p.90)
	Prolonged >0.2s.	2.15 (b)	Heart block – 📖 p.96; sick sinus syndrome, drugs (e.g. β-blockers, digoxin)
Abnormal Q–T interval	Prolonged Q–T interval	2.16 (a)	↓K⁺, drugs (e.g. TCAs, phenothiazines, amiodarone), SAH or CVA, hypothermia
	Shortened Q–T interval	2.16 (b)	↑Ca²⁺, digoxin
Abnormal P waves	↑P wave amplitude (>2.5mm)	2.17 (a)	Right atrial overload – tricuspid stenosis, pulmonary hypertension, pulmonary stenosis
	Biphasic P wave in V1 ±broad (>0.12s) often notched P wave in ≥1 limb lead	2.17 (b) & (c)	Left atrial abnormality – mitral stenosis, aortic stenosis, conduction abnormalities
Left bundle branch block (LBBB)*	QRS >0.12s. wide. Last peak is below the isoelectric line in V1	2.18 📖 p.48	IHD, ↑BP, cardiomyopathy, aortic valve disease, SVT. Artificial pacemakers may produce a similar QRS complex
Right bundle branch block (RBBB)	QRS >0.12s. wide. Last peak is above the isoelectric line in V1	2.19 📖 p.48	May be normal; congenital heart disease (e.g. ASD), valvular heart disease, IHD, pulmonary hypertension, during SVT
Incomplete bundle branch block	QRS < 0.12s with abnormal shaped QRS complex	N/A	As for RBBB or LBBB

* No comment can be made about ST segment or T wave if LBBB.

(contd. on p.50)

🛈 Always compare with previous ECGs if available.

Figure 2.14 Rate and rhythm

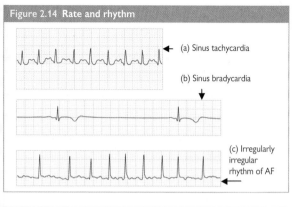

(a) Sinus tachycardia

(b) Sinus bradycardia

(c) Irregularly irregular rhythm of AF

Figure 2.15 P–R interval abnormalities

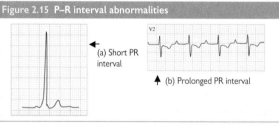

(a) Short PR interval

(b) Prolonged PR interval

Figure 2.16 Q–T interval abnormalities

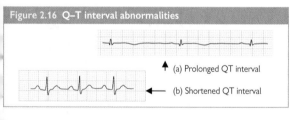

(a) Prolonged QT interval

(b) Shortened QT interval

Figure 2.17 Abnormal P waves

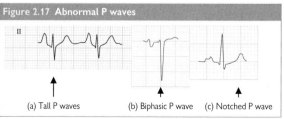

(a) Tall P waves (b) Biphasic P wave (c) Notched P wave

Figure 2.15 is reproduced from Morris F, Edhouse J, Brady W, and Camm J, (2002), The *ABC of Clinical Electrocardiography*, with permission from Blackwell BMJ Books.

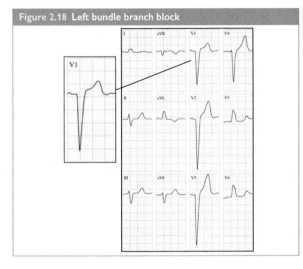

Figure 2.18 Left bundle branch block

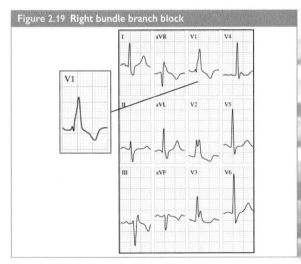

Figure 2.19 Right bundle branch block

Figures 2.18 and 2.19 are reproduced from Morris F, Edhouse J, Brady W, and Camm J, (2002), The *ABC of Clinical Electrocardiography*, with permission from Blackwell BMJ Books.

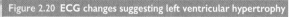

Figure 2.20 ECG changes suggesting left ventricular hypertrophy

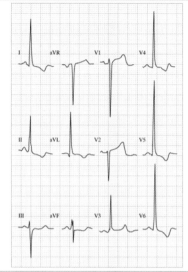

GP Notes: Scoring system for left ventricular hypertrophy (LVH)

ECG feature	Points
Amplitude – any of the following:	3
• Largest R or S wave in limb leads ≥20mm	
• S wave in leads V1 or V2 ≥30mm	
• R wave in leads V5 or V6 ≥30mm	
ST–T wave changes typical for LVH in the absence of digitalis	3
Left atrial involvement	3
Left axis deviation	2
QRS duration of ≥0.09s.	1
Delayed ventricular action time in leads V5 and V6 of ≥0.05s.	1

LVH is suggested if points total ≥5

Figure 2.20 and the above GP Notes are reproduced from Morris F, Edhouse J, Brady W, and Camm J, (2002), The *ABC of Clinical Electrocardiography*, with permission from Blackwell BMJ Books.

Table 2.8 Common ECG abnormalities and their causes (contd.)

ECG abnormality		Figure	Possible causes
Left ventricular hypertrophy (LVH)	Strain pattern – ST↓ and T wave ↓ in leads V4–6. Large voltages of QRS complex – sum of S in V1 and R in V5 or V6 alone >35mm	2.20 📖 p.49	↑BP, aortic stenosis, coarctation of the aorta, HOCM
Right ventricular hypertrophy (RVH)	Strain pattern – ST depression and T-wave inversion in leads V1–3. Dominant R in V1 with narrow QRS	2.21	Pulmonary stenosis, mitral stenosis pulmonary hypertension, ASD (±RBBB). Similar changes seen with inferior MI (T wave upright); WPW syndrome
Right axis deviation	📖 p.44	N/A	RVH/strain (e.g. following PE), cor pulmonale, pulmonary stenosis. Alone with normal QRS = left posterior hemiblock
Left axis deviation	📖 p.44	N/A	LVH/strain (e.g. ↑BP, aortic stenosis, HOCM), VSD, ASD. If occurs alone with normal QRS = left anterior hemiblock
Poor R-wave progression	Small or absent R waves up to the mid pre-cordial leads	2.22 (a)	L or R ventricular enlargement, LBBB, left pneumothorax, dextrocardia, COPD
	Reversed R-wave progression – ↓ in R-wave amplitude from V1 → mid/lateral pre-cordial leads	N/A	Right ventricular enlargement
Abnormal Q waves	>25% of succeeding R wave and/or >0.04s. wide	2.23 (b)	Normal; left pneumothorax, dextrocardia, MI; myocarditis, hyperkalaemia, cardiomyopathy, amyloid; sarcoid, scleroderma, LVH, RVH, LBBB, WPW syndrome
ST elevation	ST segment raised >1mm above baseline	2.23 (a)	MI, Prinzmetal angina, pericarditis, ventricular aneurysm
ST depression	ST segment lowered >0.5mm below baseline	2.23 (b)	Angina, ventricular strain, drugs (digoxin, verapamil), ↑K⁺, myocarditis, cardiomyopathy, fibrosis
T-wave inversion	Abnormal if inverted in leads I, II or V4–6	2.24 (a)	MI (inverts <24h. after MI); ventricular strain (see above); PE (III); digoxin (V5-6)
U waves	↑ amplitude >1mm	2.24 (b)	Drugs (e.g. quinidine, procainamide, disopyramide) or ↓K⁺
Inversion in the precordial leads		N/A	Subtle sign of ischaemia

ⓘ Always compare with previous ECGs if available.

Figure 2.21 Right ventricular hypertrophy

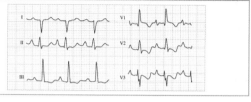

Figure 2.22 Poor R-wave progression and abnormal Q waves

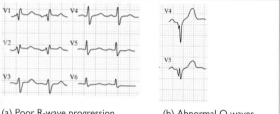

(a) Poor R-wave progression

(b) Abnormal Q waves

Figure 2.23 ST segment changes

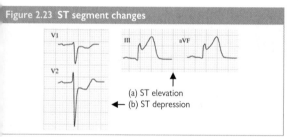

(a) ST elevation

(b) ST depression

Figure 2.24 T-wave inversion and U waves

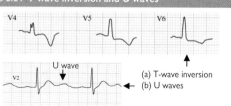

U wave

(a) T-wave inversion

(b) U waves

Figure 2.21 is reproduced from Morris F, Edhouse J, Brady W, and Camm J, (2002), The *ABC of Clinical Electrocardiography*, with permission from Blackwell BMJ Books.

24h./ambulatory ECG: ECG monitoring equipment is worn for 24h. Continuous monitoring may detect intermittent arrhythmias or ischaemia.

Exercise ECG[£]: ECG testing whilst the patient undergoes graded exercise on a treadmill/exercise bicycle. Local referral criteria vary.

Uses
● Diagnosis of ischaemic heart disease – 75% have a +ve test. There is a false +ve rate of ~5%
● Assessment of exercise tolerance
● Response to treatment
● As a prognostic indicator
● Assessment of exercise-related arrhythmias
● As a guide to rehabilitation following acute myocardial infarction
● Risk stratification in patients with HOCM
● Assessment of need for further investigation

Bruce protocol: Exercise testing is usually carried out according to a standardised protocol (standard Bruce or modified Bruce), which gradually increases the speed and gradient of the bicycle or treadmill. A number of parameters are assessed during the test:
● ECG changes
● Appearance of the patient
● Recurrence of symptoms
● BP and heart rate response.

Contraindications
● Recent MI (<7d.)
● Unstable angina
● Electrolyte disturbance
● Aortic stenosis
● Severe heart failure
● Known left main coronary artery stenosis
● LBBB (may not be possible to interpret the trace)
● Acute systemic illness
● Uncontrolled hypertension
● Acute pericarditis or myocarditis

🔔 Exercise testing carries a mortality of ~1:10,000.

Further information
BMJ Hill and Timmis *ABC of clinical electrocardiography: exercise tolerance testing* (2002) **324** p.1084–1087 (also available from 🖥 www.bmj.com)
Lancet Ashley *et al. Exercise testing in clinical medicine* (2000) **35** p.1592–1597

GMS contract			
CHD 2	% of patients with newly diagnosed angina (after 01.04.2003) who are referred for exercise testing and/or specialist assessment	7 points	40–90%
AF 2	% of patients with AF diagnosed after 01.04.2006 with ECG or specialist confirmed diagnosis	10 points	40–90%

Other cardiovascular investigations

Cardiac enzymes: Biochemical blood assay of molecules released when the heart is damaged. Used in diagnosis of MI.

- **Troponins T and I:** Preferred markers as more sensitive/specific than CK, AST or LDH. Together with CK, earliest to ↑ after MI.
- **Creatine kinase (CK):** ↑ in MI, muscle damage e.g. prolonged running or seizures, after IM injection, and with dermatomyositis (e.g. due to statins). CK–MB assay may help clarify whether a cardiac event has occurred <48h. previously.
- **Aspartate-amino transferase (AST):** ↑ in MI after CK but before LDH (below). Other causes of ↑ AST include: liver disease (suggesting hepatocyte damage), skeletal muscle damage and haemolysis.
- **Lactate dehydrogenase (LDH):** Last cardiac enzyme to be elevated. Other causes of ↑ LDH include: liver disease (suggest hepatocyte damage); haemolysis, PE, tumour necrosis.

Colour flow doppler/duplex scanning: Uses ultrasound to assess blood vessels and blood flow within them. It is a hazard-free, non invasive test and the procedure of choice for assessment/monitoring of abdominal aortic aneurysms, monitoring of peripheral arterial bypass grafts and assessing carotid stenosis in patients who have a history of stroke/TIA and might be suitable for carotid endarterectomy.

Echocardiogram (Echo): Heart ultrasound scan. Of particular value in the assessment of ventricular function, valvular heart disease and congenital heart disease. Local referral procedures vary.

2-dimensional: Produces a fan-shaped, cross-sectional, moving, real time image of the heart (Figure 2.25). May be transthoracic or trans oesophageal. Used to assess:

- Valvular abnormalities and prosthetic heart valves
- Aortic aneurysm/dissection
- Heart failure
- Pericardial effusion
- Masses within the heart
- Myocardial abnormalities (e.g. aneurysms, hypertrophy)
- Ischaemic heart disease
- Congenital heart disease.

M-mode: Plotted on a scrolling screen (Figure 2.26). Stationary structures appear as straight lines across the screen; moving structures appear as undulating lines. Usually displayed with an ECG trace to enable identification of phases of the cardiac cycle. Used to investigate movement of individual structural elements e.g. valves, chamber walls.

Doppler: Enables flow across valves and ASD/VSDs to be quantified. Colour doppler flow mapping is created by colour-encoding pulsed-wave doppler information. High blood flow velocities produce more intense colours. The display produced is then overlaid onto the 2-dimensional structural echocardiogram (Figure 2.26).

Figure 2.25 2-dimensional and M-mode echocardiogram

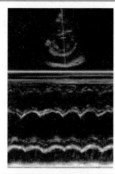

Figure 2.26 Colour doppler flow mapping showing flow through a heart valve

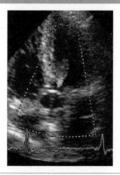

GMS contract

HF 2	% of patients with diagnosis of heart failure (diagnosed after 01.04.2006) which has been confirmed by an echocardiogram or by specialist assessment	6 points	40–90%

Angiography: Angiography remains the gold standard for 'mapping' the circulation. It is used for assessing the peripheral vasculature and the coronary arteries.

Peripheral angiography: Used for:
- Assessment of intermittent claudication and rest pain
- Diagnosis and quantification of peripheral arterial disease
- Assessment of abdominal aortic aneurysm and other peripheral arterial aneurysms.

Complications: Complication rate is 2–3% in lower limb studies. Complications include: haemorrhage, false aneurysm formation, arterial thrombosis and peripheral embolization.

Digital subtraction angiography (DSA): Images before and after introduction of contrast medium are stored digitally. They are then processed electronically and the 'before' and 'after' images subtracted from each other to eliminate the images of everything except the contrast filled arteries.

Cardiac catheterization: Refer via 2° care. Involves passing a catheter, usually via the femoral or brachial artery, to the heart.

Coronary angiography: The vast majority of patients who undergo cardiac catheterization have coronary angiography – usually in conjunction with left heart catheterization. Indications include:
- Diagnosis of coronary artery disease
- Assessment of angina uncontrolled by medication
- Assessment of suitability for coronary intervention
- Recurrence of angina following coronary angioplasty or bypass grafting
- A strongly positive exercise test.

Severity of coronary narrowing is described using percentage stenosis – >50% is usually regarded as significant.

Other indications for cardiac catheterization
- To measure pressures within the heart and great vessels
- To assess oxygen saturation via blood samples
- To assess arrhythmic foci
- To perform intravascular ultrasound
- To perform other procedures e.g. angioplasty, valvuloplasty, cardiac biopsy

Complications
- Haemorrhage at the site of insertion (0.56%)
- Arrhythmia (0.56%)
- MI (0.07%)
- Stroke (0.07%) or thromboembolism elsewhere
- Trauma to the heart or blood vessels
- Infection
- Death (0.14%)

Radionucleotide imaging: Refer via 2° care. Involves IV administration of a γ-emitting radionucleotide and gamma camera monitoring.
- *Radionucleotide angiography:* Uses technetium[99m]-labelled RBCs to calculate left ventricular ejection fraction and assess ventricular action.
- *Myocardial perfusion scintigraphy:* Uses thallium[201] injected IV during exercise testing to demonstrate areas of poorly perfused myocardium.

Cardiac MRI/magnetic resonance angiography: Used increasingly in 2° care to provide detailed structural information about the heart and rapid angiographic images.

Advice for patients: Information for patients about cardiac investigations

British Heart Foundation ☎ 0845 0708 070 🖥 www.bhf.org.uk

Chapter 3

Diagnosis and management of cardiac and vascular problems in primary care

Prevention of cardiovascular disease

Coronary heart disease (CHD) is the most common cause of death in UK (1:4 deaths). Mortality is falling but morbidity rising.

Primary prevention: *Objective:* To stop cardiovascular disease (CVD) developing in a population.

Strategies:

- **Population strategy:** Influences the factors which ↑ risk of CVD in an entire population e.g. anti-smoking campaigns. GPs can do this by displaying health education posters/literature where all patients have access (waiting room, practice leaflet).
- **High-risk strategy:** Identifies individuals at high risk and attempts to ↓ their risk. Selection of patients is based on overall risk. High risk patients are those with DM and otherwise apparently healthy individuals at high risk of developing symptomatic atherosclerotic disease (CVD risk of ≥20% over 10y.) Risk can be estimated using tables (📖 p.154–5). Even though plans have been announced to introduce 'health checks' for all at key points throughout life, only small benefit is gained by screening an entire population and population screening is not cost-effective[R]. An opportunistic strategy targeting high-risk individuals is preferable.

Secondary prevention: *Objective:* To stop progression of symptomatic CVD. 46% people who die from MI are already known to have CVD. There is strong evidence that targeting patients with CVD for risk factor modification is effective in ↓ risk of recurrent CVD[S].

The GP's role: GPs have a role in:

- Identification of patients who would benefit from 1° prevention through opportunistic risk factor screening or routine checks (e.g. new patient checks)[£]. Quality and outcome framework points (and thus payments) are available for doing this
- Ensuring patients who have proven atherosclerotic disease have ongoing follow-up (through disease registers, routine recall and follow-up by the practice, PCO and/or 2° care services, and monitoring of drug prescriptions). Points gained for meeting secondary prevention targets contained within the quality and outcome framework reward practices for secondary prevention
- Promoting lifestyle modification in at-risk patients[£]
- Ensuring current best care guidelines are followed and treatment regimes are updated as policies change
- Checking the process through audit.

Further information

DoH National Service Framework: Coronary heart disease (2000 and update 2005) 🖥 www.dh.gov.uk
SIGN 🖥 www.sign.ac.uk
Risk estimation and the prevention of cardiovascular disease (2007)
JBS2: Joint British Societies' Guidelines on prevention of cardiovascular disease in clinical practice. *Heart* (2005). **91** (Supp. 5): V1–52.
NICE MI: Secondary prevention (2007). 🖥 www.nice.org.uk

Table 3.1 Risk factors for heart disease

Non-modifiable	Modifiable (proven benefit)	Modifiable (unproven benefit)
Age – ↑ with age	Smoking – 🕮 p.188	Haemostatic factors – ↑ plasma fibrinogen
Sex – ♂>♀ in those <65y.	Hyperlipidaemia – 🕮 p.182	Apolipoproteins – ↑ Lipoprotein(a)
Ethnic origin – in the UK people who originate from the Indian subcontinent have ↑ risk, Afro-Caribbeans have ↓ risk	Hypertension – 🕮 p.168	Homocysteine – ↑ blood homocysteine
	DM – 🕮 p.162	
	Diet – 🕮 p.72	Vitamin levels – ↓ blood folate, vitamin B₁₂ and B₆
Socio-economic position	Obesity – 🕮 p.192	
Personal history of CHD	Physical inactivity – 🕮 p.198	Depression
Family history of CHD – <55y. ♂; <65y. ♀	Left ventricular dysfunction/heart failure (2° prevention) – 🕮 p.76	
Low birth weight (IUGR)	Coronary prone behaviour – competitiveness, aggression and feeling under time pressure (2° prevention) – behaviour modification is associated with ↓ risk	

GMS contract

Primary prevention

Records 11	BP of patients aged ≥45y. is recorded in the preceding 5y. for ≥65% of patients	10 points	
Records 17	BP of patients aged ≥45y. is recorded in the preceding 5y. for ≥80% of patients	5 points	
Records 22	% of patients aged >15y. whose notes record smoking status in the past 27mo., except those who have never smoked where smoking status need be recorded only once	11 points	40–90%
Information 5	The practice supports smokers in stopping smoking by a strategy which includes providing literature and offering appropriate therapy	2 points	

Secondary prevention of cardiovascular disease: 🕮 p.65

Advice for patients: Information for patients on coronary prevention

British Heart Foundation ☎ 0845 0708 070 🖥 www.bhf.org.uk

Angina

Affects ~2% population in UK. Incidence ↑ with age. ♂>♀. Coronary artery disease is the most common cause. Rarer causes include HOCM valve disease, hypoperfusion during arrhythmia, arteritis, anaemia or thyrotoxicosis. Mortality (usually sudden death or after MI or acute LVF) is ~0.5–4%/y. – doubled if co-existent left ventricular dysfunction.

Presentation of stable angina: Diagnosis is usually made on history:
- *Pain:* Episodic central-crushing or band-like chest pain which may radiate → jaw/neck and/or 1 or both arms. Pain in the arms/neck may be the only symptom. Ask about frequency, severity, duration and timing of attacks.
- *Precipitating/relieving factors:* Precipitated by exertion, cold, emotion and/or heavy meals. Pain stops with rest or GTN spray.
- *Associated symptoms:* May be associated with palpitations, sweating, nausea and/or breathlessness during attacks.
- *Presence of risk factors:* Smoking history; family history; history of other vascular disease e.g. CVA/TIA, peripheral vascular disease.

Examination: There are usually no physical signs though anaemia may exacerbate symptoms. Check BMI and BP. Look for murmurs (especially ejection systolic murmur of aortic stenosis) and evidence of peripheral vascular disease and carotid bruits (especially in diabetics).

First-line investigations
- *Blood:* FBC, fasting lipid profile, fasting blood glucose. Consider checking ESR (to exclude arteritis) and TFTs if clinical suspicion of thyrotoxicosis.
- *12-lead resting ECG:* Provides information on rhythm, presence of heart block, previous MI, myocardial hypertrophy and/or ischaemia.

⚠ A normal ECG does not exclude coronary artery disease, but an abnormal ECG identifies those at higher risk of cardiac events in the next year – consider referral for further investigation.

Differential diagnosis: Chest pain – 📖 p.39

Prinzmetal (variant) angina: Angina at rest due to coronary artery spasm. ECG shows ST elevation.

Management: Refer to cardiology to exclude MI and atherosclerotic angina. GTN alleviates immediate episodes. Calcium-channel blockers are used to prevent angina.

Unstable angina: Pain on minimal or no exertion, pain at rest (may occur at night) or angina which is rapidly worsening in intensity, frequency or duration. *Incidence:* 6/10,000/y.; 15% suffer MI in <1mo.

Management: Urgent referral to cardiology. Treat as for acute MI and admit if attacks are severe, occur at rest or last >20min. even with GTN spray – 📖 p.68.

Advice for patients: Information for patients

British Heart Foundation ☎ 0845 0708 070 🖳 www.bhf.org.uk

Further information
SIGN Management of stable angina (2007) 🖳 www.sign.ac.uk
Cardiac rehabilitation 🖳 www.cardiacrehabilitation.org.uk

Management of stable angina

General advice
- *Driving:* Patients who drive should inform the DVLA and their insurance company of the diagnosis. Vocational drivers – 📖 p.222.
- *Occupation:* Patients may not be able to undertake heavy work – give advice and support. Special rules apply to some occupations e.g. merchant seamen, airline pilots – advise patients to consult their occupational health department.

Non-drug treatment[£]: Aimed at 2° prevention of CHD:
- *Smoking cessation* – 📖 p.188
- *Hypertension* – Check BP and, always treat ≥140/85 – 📖 p.168
- *Diet* – Advise healthy diet (oily fish, low cholesterol, ↑ fruit and vegetables, ↓ salt) and, if obese, aim to ↓ weight until BMI <25 (📖 p.192)
- *Alcohol* – ↓ excess consumption. *Targets:* <3u/d. ♂; <2u/d. ♀
- *Exercise* – ↑ aerobic exercise within the limits set by the disease state
- *Diabetes* – Treat any underlying DM – 📖 p.162
- *Cardiac rehabilitation* – May be helpful for patients with stable angina or after surgery/percutaneous coronary revascularization.

Drug treatment: 📖 p.66

Referral for exercise ECG[£]: 📖 p.52. Refer all patients with angina (unless contraindicated) to allow risk stratification. Advise patients to take their usual medication prior to going for the test.

Contraindications
- Symptoms uncontrolled by maximal medical treatment
- Uncertain diagnosis
- Proven or suspected aortic stenosis or cardiomyopathy or physically incapable of performing the test for reasons other than angina
- Results of stress testing would not affect management
- LBBB on ECG

⚠ If contraindicated refer to cardiology.

Referral to cardiology: E=Admit; U=Urgent; S=Soon; R=Routine
- Unstable angina/rapidly progressive symptoms – E
- Aortic stenosis with angina – U
- Angina following MI – U/S
- Abnormal ECG at diagnosis – U/S
- Angina not controlled by medication – U/S/R
- If diagnosis is in doubt – S/R
- Exercise test contraindicated – R
- Strong family history – R
- Other factors e.g. occupation affected – R

⚠ Many hospitals now run open-access chest pain clinics.

Bypass surgery (CABG) and angioplasty
Both percutaneous coronary revascularization (angioplasty ± stenting) and CABG ↓ symptoms in 80–90%. Compared to medical therapy they do not ↓ MI/mortality unless severe left main coronary artery disease or 2-/3- vessel disease + left ventricular dysfunction, when CABG ↑ survival.

GMS contract			
CHD 1	The practice can produce a register of patients with coronary heart disease	4 points	
CHD 2	% of patients with newly diagnosed angina (after 01.04.2003) who are referred for exercise testing and/or specialist assessment	up to 7 points	40–90%
CHD 5	% of patients with coronary heart disease whose notes have a record of BP in the previous 15mo.	up to 7 points	40–90%
CHD 6	% of patients with coronary heart disease in whom the last BP reading (measured in the last 15mo.) is ≤150/90	up to 19 points	40–70%
CHD 7	% of patients with coronary heart disease whose notes have a record of total cholesterol in the previous 15mo.	up to 7 points	40–90%
CHD 8	% of patients with coronary heart disease whose last measured total cholesterol (measured in the last 15mo.) is ≤5mmol/l	up to 17 points	40–70%
CHD 9	% of patients with coronary heart disease with a record in the last 15mo. that aspirin, an alternative antiplatelet therapy or an anticoagulant is being taken (unless a contraindication or side-effects are recorded)	up to 7 points	40–90%
CHD 10	% of patients with coronary heart disease who are currently treated with a β-blocker (unless a contraindication or side-effects are recorded)	up to 7 points	40–60%
CHD 11	% of patients with a history of myocardial infarction (diagnosed after 01.04.2003) who are currently treated with an ACE inhibitor or angiotensin II antagonist	up to 7 points	40–80%
CHD 12	% of patients with coronary heart disease who have a record of influenza immunization in the preceding 1st September–31st March	up to 7 points	40–90%
Depression 1	% of patients on the CHD register for whom case finding for depression has been undertaken in the previous 15mo. using the 2 standard screening questions (📖 p.248)	up to 8 points	40–90%
Smoking 1	% of patients with any/combination of coronary heart disease, stroke or TIA, hypertension, diabetes, COPD or asthma whose notes record smoking status in the previous 15mo. Except those who have never smoked where smoking status need only be recoreded once since diagnosis	up to 33 points	40–90%
Smoking 2	% of patients with any or a combination of the conditions listed in 'smoking 1' who smoke whose notes contain a record that smoking cessation advice or referral to a specialist service, where available, has been offered within the previous 15mo.	up to 35 points	40–90%

Heart failure: 📖 p.247   **Hypertension:** 📖 p.253   **Diabetes:** 📖 p.255

Drug treatment of angina

Symptom control: *BNF 2.6*

As required medication
- Glyceryl trinitrate (GTN) spray is used for 'as required' symptom relief for angina.
- If symptoms are infrequent (≤2 attacks/wk.) GTN may be used alone; if attacks are more frequent add regular symptomatic treatment (below).
- Advise 1–2 puffs as needed in response to pain and before engaging in activities that bring on pain.
- If response to GTN spray is poor, consider a buccal preparation.

ⓘ Sublingual GTN tablets are an alternative to GTN spray but deteriorate after 8wk.

⚠ Warn patients to call for help (dial 999 or ring emergency GP) if chest pain lasts >20min. despite GTN spray.

Regular treatment
- If symptoms are severe or >2x/wk., prescribe regular symptomatic treatment – Table 3.2.
- Introduce medication in a stepwise manner according to response:
  - Start with a β-blocker (e.g atenolol 50–100mg od) unless contraindicated/intolerant.
  - Add a long-acting dihydropyridine calcium-channel blocker (e.g. amlodipine 5mg od) as 2nd line.
  - Add a long-acting nitrate (e.g. isosorbide mononitrate 20mg bd/tds) as 3rd line.
  - For patients without left ventricular dysfunction and in whom β-blockers are inappropriate, use diltiazem (60mg bd/tds) or verapamil (80–120mg tds) as 1st line treatment and add a long-acting nitrate if symptom control is not adequate.
  - For patients with left ventricular dysfunction, use a long-acting nitrate as 1st line treatment and add a long-acting dihydropyridine calcium-channel blocker if symptom control is not adequate.
  - For those intolerant of standard treatment, or where standard treatment has failed, try nicorandil (5–10mg bd).
- Within any drug class use the cheapest preparation that the patient can tolerate, will comply with, and which controls symptoms.

⚠ Avoid combination of β-blockers and rate-limiting calcium-channel blockers (verapamil, diltiazem) due to risk of bradycardia/asystole.

2° prevention

Aspirin: ↓ mortality by 34%. Unless contraindicated, give 75mg od to all patients with angina. Consider clopidogrel 75mg od if aspirin intolerant.

Statins: ↓ in total cholesterol and LDL by 25–35% using statin therapy → ↓ CHD mortality by 25–35%[S]. Trial data suggest *all* patients with proven CHD benefit from ↓ in total cholesterol and LDL, irrespective of initial cholesterol concentration[S] – 🕮 p.186.

Table 3.2 Drug treatment of angina

Drug	Treatment notes
β-blockers *BNF 2.4* ⚠ May accumulate in patients with renal failure – ↓ dose.	Effective for symptom control and to prevent vascular events. If left ventricular dysfunction, introduce with caution if no evidence of active heart failure (↓ mortality) Check fully β-blocked by monitoring heart rate – resting heart rate ≤65bpm; post-exercise (e.g. walking up 2 flights of stairs) heart rate ≤90bpm. Further increases in dose once adequately β-blocked are usually unhelpful. *Side-effects:* cold extremities and sleep disturbances, lethargy and bradycardia are relatively common. ⚠ Warn patients not to stop suddenly or run out. If the patient needs to stop the drug, tail off over 4wk. *Contraindications:* asthma, bradycardia.
Dihydropyridine calcium-channel blockers *BNF 2.6.2*	Amlodipine, felodipine, isradipine, lacidipine, lercanidipine, nicardipine, nifedipine, nimodipine and nisoldipine All equally effective in symptom control. No evidence of cardioprotective effect. *Side-effects:* headache, nausea, flushing and peripheral oedema especially. *Contraindications:* vary. Don't use if aortic stenosis, <1mo. post-MI or uncontrolled heart failure except with specialist advice.
Rate-limiting calcium-channel blockers *BNF 2.6.2*	Diltiazem and verapamil *Side-effects:* headache, nausea, flushing and peripheral oedema especially. *Contraindications:* avoid in patients with heart block or heart failure. Do not combine with β-blockers.
Long-acting nitrates *BNF 2.6.1* e.g. isosorbide mononitrate (ISMO)	Oral and patch preparations (dosages ≥ 10mg/24h.) are available. Start with a low dose and ↑ as tolerated. Side-effects are common. *Side-effects:* headache, postural hypotension and dizziness – wear off with use. Reflex tachycardia may ↓ coronary blood flow and worsen angina. *Tolerance:* many patients rapidly develop tolerance with ↓ therapeutic effect. To avoid this allow a nitrate-free period of 4–8h./d. overnight by removing patches at night or giving the 2nd dose of ISMO at 4p.m. *Contraindications:* HOCM, aortic stenosis, constrictive pericarditis, mitral stenosis, severe anaemia, closed-angle glaucoma.
Potassium channel activator *BNF 2.6.3*	Nicorandil Similar efficacy to other anti-anginal drugs in controlling symptoms. May produce additional symptomatic benefit in combination with other anti-anginal drugs (unlicensed). Headache is common – usually transitory. *Contraindications:* left ventricular failure, hypotension.

Myocardial infarct

⚠️ Diagnosis is sometimes not obvious: always have a high index of suspicion. It is also difficult to tell the difference between acute myocardial infarct (MI) and unstable angina in general practice. Treat as for acute MI.

Typical presentation: Sustained central chest pain not relieved by sublingual GTN.

Other features that may be present
- Collapse ± cardiac arrest
- Breathlessness
- Anxiety/fear of dying
- Nausea ± vomiting
- Sweating
- Pain in 1 or both arms, jaw, back or upper abdomen.

ℹ️ May occasionally be silent especially in patients with DM.

Examination: Pulse, BP, JVP, heart sounds, chest (?pulmonary oedema)

Investigation: *ECG* – ST elevation (Figure 3.1) *or* R waves and ST depression in leads V1–V3 (posterior infarction) *or* new LBBB.

Action:

When the call for assistance is made:
If MI is suspected, arrange immediate transfer to hospital – for thrombolysis to be effective it must be given as soon as possible after the onset of pain. Seeing the patient before arranging transfer introduces unnecessary delays.

If possible attend the patient once the ambulance has been called to assist – there is a lot a GP can do that an ambulance crew cannot. If the patient is seen:
- Give aspirin 300mg po (unless contraindicated).
- Insert IV cannula.
- Give IV analgesia (diamorphine 2.5–5mg). Repeat in 15min. as necessary.
- Give IV antiemetic (metoclopramide 10mg).
- Give sublingual GTN to act as a coronary artery vasodilator (if systolic BP >90 and pulse <100bpm).
- If available give oxygen.
- If bradycardia, give atropine 300mcgm IV and further doses of 300mcgm if needed to a maximum of 1.2mg.

Thrombolysis in general practice: May be appropriate in places where transfer to hospital takes >½ h. Special training and equipment is necessary.

Follow-up care: 📖 p.72

- *If the patient is seen <24h. after an acute episode* – admit for specialist assessment.
- *If the patient is seen >24h. after an acute episode, but still has residual pain or other symptoms* – admit.
- *If the patient is seen >24h. after an acute episode and is well* – start regular aspirin, supply with GTN spray, warn what to do if any further episodes of acute chest pain and follow up as for MI post-discharge (📖 p.72).

Figure 3.1 Sequence of ECG changes after MI

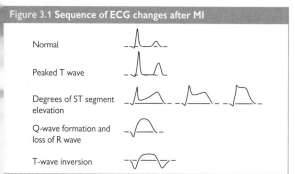

Normal	
Peaked T wave	
Degrees of ST segment elevation	
Q-wave formation and loss of R wave	
T-wave inversion	

Figure 3.1 is reproduced from Morris F, Edhouse J, Brady W, and Camm J, (2002), The *ABC of Clinical Electrocardiography*, with permission from Blackwell BMJ Books.

Advice for patients: Patient experiences of heart attack

Having a heart attack

'It was totally out of the blue. I was sitting down, I'd had breakfast, and I was just thinking about making a cup of coffee, and suddenly this sort of pain hit me. And initially I thought, well it might be indigestion or something, but it went on, and after I would guess 10 or 15 seconds, it was so excruciating.

I'd never experienced a pain like this, it was just coming in waves… [my family] called an ambulance probably within two or three minutes. And this pain…wouldn't go away and basically it was so excruciating … I think I probably realised I'd had a heart attack. I had a sort of tingling sense in my right arm.'

'I first suspected there was something wrong when I thought I had a bad bout of indigestion…I thought that I would sleep it off. My wife gave me some indigestion pills that she said were very effective. But in the early hours of the morning I realised that it wasn't getting any better. She phoned the surgery when she could and booked an appointment….

Going back upstairs after a shower, it really hit me. So she phoned them … They asked her for symptoms and she said, "Well he's got this pain in his arm," which meant nothing to us. It meant nothing to me, I thought I'd strained a muscle chopping the tree down, and they said, "There's an ambulance on it's way," and I was taken to hospital.'

Coming home after a heart attack

'On the day I was discharged, I went for a short walk … down the corridor, down to the bottom of the hospital to the newsagent's. I felt a bit shaky then because I wasn't used to walking because it had knocked the stuffing out of me a bit. So I realised I was going to have to take it really easy for the next few days, few weeks even… I just did everything at a slower pace, taking my time. Gradually I was building up until I could do more and more.'

'So I was in hospital 10 days and did a successful treadmill, which is sort of a passport to get out really … and went home. You immediately feel very inadequate at home.'

Reaction of others

'So I think people thought that, you know, I should behave like an invalid perhaps, or they should try to wrap me in cotton wool a bit. You know with the best of intentions, but people don't know what having a heart attack is like so they don't really know how to treat you afterwards.'

'Of course [my wife] was anxious as well when I got home because it was all down to her then, which was worrying, and she wouldn't let me do a thing, which was very frustrating.

You know I mean, hospital's all on one level. Obviously we've got stairs here. She said, "No, you're only walking up the stairs once. Don't come up and down two or three times for this and that, you're going to bed. You're just going to tackle the stairs once a day," and this sort of thing.

And I thought, "well that's ridiculous because I certainly felt a lot stronger than that." But, well, I try to do as I'm told [laughs]. It isn't easy.

'But the person it affected most was my wife. She took a long time to sort of release the apron strings…it's had more of an effect on my family, I think, than it has on me.'

Information needs

'So he sat down with us for nearly an hour, talking about diet and lifestyle, exercise, sort of doing things gradually, but mainly the fact that there's no reason why I couldn't get back to as normal a life as possible…He explained that I'd be on medication…But he talked very much about taking control, that you can do this, you can do that. You can stop eating red meat, you can stop smoking. You can start walking as soon as we tell you to, to build up, you can join the gym, you can look at what other foods are healthy. It was all very positive about taking control and sort of getting your life back.'

'And you pick up every leaflet about heart attacks and look up things on the internet about angiograms and stents, but that's like empowerment. It means that you know this heart attack struck you down, but now you're going to do something about stopping having another one.'

Information for patients

British Heart Foundation ☎ 0845 0708 070 🖳 www.bhf.org.uk
DIPEx Database of personal and health experiences: heart attack 🖳 www.dipex.org

After myocardial infarction

Modification of risk factors

- *Cholesterol:* Aim to ↓ total cholesterol by 25% or to <4mmol/L – whichever is the lower value, *or* ↓ LDL cholesterol by 30% or to <2.0mmol/L – whichever is the lower value, using statin therapy → ↓ CHD mortality by 25–35%[S]. All patients with proven CHD benefit from ↓ in total cholesterol and LDL irrespective of initial cholesterol concentration[G] – 📖 p.186.
- *Smoking cessation:* 📖 p.188. ↓ risk of death by 50% over 15y.
- *Hypertension:* Check BP and always treat if ≥140/85 – 📖 p.168.
- *Diet:* Advise healthy diet (low cholesterol, ↑ fruit and vegetables, ↓ salt) and, if obese, aim to ↓ weight until BMI <25. Diets rich in omega-6 and omega-3 fatty acids (found in oily fish, vegetables and nuts) ↓ CHD in 2° prevention through ↓ in risk of thrombosis. Consider providing supplements if MI <3mo. previously and dietary deficiency.
- *Alcohol:* ↓ excess consumption. *Targets:* <3u/d. ♂; <2u/d. ♀.
- *Exercise:* ↑ aerobic exercise within the limits set by the disease state.
- *Diabetes:* Treat any underlying DM – 📖 p.162.
- *Reinforce information* given during cardiac rehabilitation.

⚠ Serum cholesterol levels ↓ after MI and remain ↓ for several weeks.

β-blockers: Unless contraindicated, start all patients on an oral β-blocker (e.g. atenolol) soon after MI and continue indefinitely Estimated to prevent 12 deaths/1000 treated/y.

ACE inhibitors: ↓ myocardial work and ↓ deaths within 1mo. post MI by 5/1000 treated. Survival advantage is sustained >1y. even if treatment is not continued long term. Effects are greater for patients with heart failure at presentation. **Long-term ACE inhibitors:** Trials show ↓ mortality for all patients.

Aspirin: Starting aspirin <24h. after MI prevents 80 vascular events over the next 2y./1000 patients treated. Unless contraindicated continue lifelong. There is some debate about optimal dose – usual practice is to give 75mg od from then onwards. Occasionally (e.g. left ventricular aneurysm, AF) anticoagulation is indicated.

Exercise testing: Routine exercise testing identifies those likely to have angina post-MI who might benefit from early angiography ± angioplasty or CABG.

Cardiac rehabilitation: ↓ risk of death by 20–25%. Provided by specialist multidisciplinary teams. **Components include:** psychological support, information about CHD, modification of risk factors.

Dressler syndrome (Post-MI syndrome): Develops 2–10wk after MI or heart surgery. Thought to be due to autoantibodies to heart muscle. Presents with recurrent fever and chest pain ± pleural and/or pericardial effusion.

Management: Refer urgently for cardiology/general medical advice Treatment is with steroids and NSAIDs.

See 📖 p.65 and p.245 for CHD prevention targets.

Support after discharge

Physical activity – advise gradual ↑ in activity. Ensure goals given match those given by local cardiac rehabilitation. *Guide:*
- 2wk. after MI – stroll in garden or street
- 4wk. after MI – walk ½ mile/d.
- 4–6wk. after MI – ↑ to 2 miles/d. by 6wk.
- From 6wk. – ↑ speed of walking, aim 2 miles in <30min.

Sexual activity – resume after 6wk. A leaflet is available from the British Heart Foundation.

Return to work – *guide:*
- Sedentary workers: 4–6wk. after uncomplicated MI
- Light manual workers: 6–8 wk. after uncomplicated MI
- Heavy manual workers: 3 mo. after uncomplicated MI.

Psychological effects – ≈½ are depressed 1wk. after MI and 25% after 1y. Educate about CHD. Check for depression, counsel, and treat as needed.

Driving – no driving for 1mo. after MI. Inform car insurance company but no need to inform DVLA. HGV and PSV licence holders must notify the DVLA. Driving may be allowed after assessment.

Flying – most airlines will not carry passengers for 2 wk. post-MI and then only if able to climb 1 flight of stairs without difficulty.

Ongoing follow-up

- *Monitoring health* – continue regular reviews at least annually lifelong. Check for symptoms and signs of cardiac dysfunction (breathlessness, palpitations, angina), depression, carer stress.
- *Monitoring drug therapy* – ongoing prescription of drugs, monitoring of compliance and side-effects, changing medication if clinical circumstances or best practice alter.
- *Ongoing 2° prevention through modification of risk factors.*

British Heart Foundation ☎ 0845 0708 070 🖥 www.bhf.org.uk

Further information

DoH National Service Framework: Coronary heart disease (2000) 🖥 www.dh.gov.uk

Cardiac rehabilitation 🖥 www.cardiacrehabilitation.org.uk

JBS2 Joint British Societies' guidelines on prevention of cardiovascular disease in clinical practice. *Heart* (2005): **91** (Suppl. 5); V1–52

NICE MI: Secondary prevention (2007). 🖥 www.nice.org.uk

Acute left ventricular failure (acute LVF)

Severe acute breathlessness due to pulmonary oedema. Urgent treatment is needed to save life.

Presenting features
- Sudden acute breathlessness
- Fatigue
- Cough ± haemoptysis (usually pink and frothy)
- Tends to occur at night
- Some relief gained from sitting/standing.

Signs
- Dyspnoea
- Tachycardia – gallop rhythm may be present
- Coarse, wet-sounding crackles at both bases
- Ankle/sacral oedema if right heart failure also present
- ± hypotension

Differential diagnosis: Other causes of acute breathlessness (especially asthma) – 📖 p.41.

Action
- If severe, call for ambulance support.
- Sit the patient up.
- Be reassuring – it is very frightening to be very short of breath.
- Give 100% oxygen if available and no history of COPD (24% if history of COPD).
- Give furosemide 40–80mg slowly IV (or bumetanide 1–2mg).
- Give diamorphine 2.5–5mg IV over 5min.
- Give metoclopramide 10mg IV (can be mixed with diamorphine).
- Give GTN spray, 2 puffs sublingually.

Admission: Depends on severity and cause of attack, response to treatment and social support. *Always admit if:*
- Alone at home
- Inadequate social support
- Suspected cause of acute LVF warrants admission (e.g. acute MI)
- Very breathless and no improvement over ½ h. with treatment at home
- Hypotension or arrhythmia.

Further information: Chronic heart failure – 📖 p.76.

Advice for patients: Patient experiences of acute heart failure

'On the Sunday morning I woke up and I felt quite ill. I felt a sort of crackly sound, like a crunching of crystal sound...I felt this fluidness ... in my lungs, and I had a spell of vomiting, which was a frothy fluid, and blood which was the lining of the lungs. And at the time I didn't quite understand it. Now I do know and can appreciate, it was the oedema, which was the lungs filling up with water, and that is a feeling of drowning in your own ... within your own body, which is rather frightening.'

'Well it felt as if I had a chest infection so I went to the doctor, but they couldn't hear anything on my chest at all so I was told to go away and see if it got better ... And so it didn't really get better ... I was getting puffed out walking to the car from the supermarket. I was getting puffed out walking up the stairs, but not too much at that time ... Then one night I started getting really out of breath and sort of gasping for breath, and it got worse really ... The next night I started breathing really heavily. I couldn't get my breath at all and I sat down and I tried to breathe easily, and I thought well if this a panic attack then I need to keep calm. So I tried to keep calm and I tried to breathe easily and I couldn't. And my husband came in and he didn't think that I should wait any longer and he actually called [out-of-hours service].'

75

Chronic heart failure

Chronic heart failure occurs when output of the heart is inadequate to meet the needs of the body. It is the end stage of all diseases of the heart. *Prevalence:* 3–20/1000 population (1–1.6%). Incidence ↑ with age.

Causes of chronic heart failure

High output: The heart is working at normal or ↑ rate but the needs of the body are ↑ beyond that which the heart can supply e.g. hyperthyroidism, anaemia, Paget's disease, A–V malformation.

Low output: ↓ heart function. *Causes:*
- ↑ *pre-load* e.g. mitral regurgitation, fluid overload.
- *Pump failure:*
  - Cardiac muscle disease – IHD (46%), cardiomyopathy
  - ↓ expansion of heart and restricted filling – restrictive cardiomyopathy, constrictive pericarditis, tamponade
  - Inadequate heart rate – β-blockers, heart block, post-MI
  - Arrhythmia – AF commonest, ≈30% patients with heart failure
  - ↓ power – negatively ionotropic drugs e.g. verapamil, diltiazem.
- *Chronic excessive afterload:* ↑ BP (70% – may be in combination with IHD), aortic stenosis.

Primary right heart failure: e.g. pulmonary hypertension (📖 p.86), tricuspid incompetence.

Risk factors
- Smoking
- Alcohol – toxic effect on the heart – cause of heart failure in 2–3%
- DM
- Obesity
- High total cholesterol:HDL ratio
- Left ventricular hypertrophy on echo.

Diagnosis: Clinical diagnosis is difficult. Early signs are non-specific e.g. lethargy and malaise. 20–30% patients diagnosed by their GP as having heart failure do not have any demonstrable abnormality of cardiac function on echo testing. Take a detailed history and do a clinical examination to exclude other disorders.

Algorithm for diagnosing heart failure: Figure 3.2.

Classification and symptoms

Left ventricular failure (LVF): Failure of the left ventricle, causing back pressure into the pulmonary system, and giving symptoms and signs within the respiratory system. Symptoms include:
- Shortness of breath (on exertion, orthopnoea, PND)
- ↓ exercise tolerance
- Lethargy/fatigue
- Nocturnal cough (may bring up pink froth or have haemoptysis)
- Wheeze.

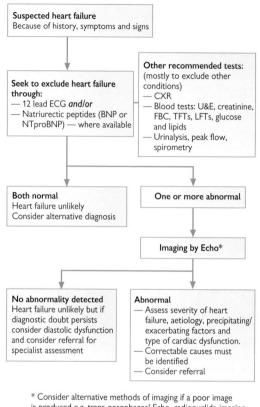

Figure 3.2 NICE algorithm for diagnosing heart failure

Suspected heart failure
Because of history, symptoms and signs

↓

Seek to exclude heart failure through:
— 12 lead ECG *and/or*
— Natriurectic peptides (BNP or NTproBNP) — where available

Other recommended tests:
(mostly to exclude other conditions)
— CXR
— Blood tests: U&E, creatinine, FBC, TFTs, LFTs, glucose and lipids
— Urinalysis, peak flow, spirometry

↓

Both normal
Heart failure unlikely
Consider alternative diagnosis

One or more abnormal

↓

Imaging by Echo*

↓

No abnormality detected
Heart failure unlikely but if diagnostic doubt persists consider diastolic dysfunction and consider referral for specialist assessment

Abnormal
— Assess severity of heart failure, aetiology, precipitating/ exacerbating factors and type of cardiac dysfunction.
— Correctable causes must be identified
— Consider referral

* Consider alternative methods of imaging if a poor image is produced e.g. trans-oesophageal Echo, radionuclide imaging or cardiac MRI.

Right ventricular failure (RVF): Failure of the right ventricle, causing back pressure into the peripheral circulation, resulting in symptoms signs in the abdomen or limbs. Symptoms include:

- Swelling of ankles (or sacrum if bedbound)
- Abdominal discomfort due to liver distention
- Nausea and anorexia
- Fatigue and wasting
- Often ↑ weight.

Congestive cardiac failure (CCF): Failure of both ventricles.

Signs

- Cachexia and muscle wasting
- ↑ respiratory rate ± cyanosis
- ↑ pulse rate
- Cardiomegaly and displaced apex beat
- Right ventricular heave
- ↑ JVP
- Pulsus alternans
- 3rd heart sound
- Basal crepitations ± pleural effusions and/or wheeze
- Pitting oedema of the ankles
- Hepatomegaly ± jaundice
- Ascites

Complications

- Arrhythmias – especially AF & VT
- Stroke or peripheral embolus
- DVT/PE
- Malabsorption
- Hepatic congestion/dysfunctio
- Muscle wasting.

Other conditions that may present with similar symptoms

- Obesity
- Respiratory disease
- Venous insufficiency in lower limbs
- Drug-induced ankle swelling (e.g. calcium-channel blockers) or fluid retention (e.g. NSAIDs)
- Hypoalbuminaemia
- Intrinsic renal or hepatic disease
- Pulmonary embolic disease
- Depression and/or anxiety
- Severe anaemia
- Thyroid disease
- Bilateral renal artery stenosis
- Intrinsic renal or hepatic disease
- Pulmonary embolic disease
- Depression and/or anxiety
- Severe anaemia or thyroid disease
- Bilateral renal artery stenosis

Table 3.3 New York Heart Association classification of heart failure according to functional limitations

Class 1	No limitation to physical activity
Class 2	Slight limitation of exercise (fatigue, dyspnoea)
Class 3	Marked limitation of activity (comfortable at rest but slight exertion causes symptoms)
Class 4	Symptoms even at rest

GMS contract

HF 1	The practice can produce a register of patients with heart failure	4 points	
HF 2	% of patients with a diagnosis of heart failure (diagnosed after 01.04.2006) which has been confirmed by an echocardiogram or by specialist assessment	6 points	40–90%
HF 3	% of patients with a current diagnosis of heart failure due to left ventricular dysfunction who are currently treated with an ACE inhibitor or Angiotensin Receptor Blocker, who can tolerate therapy and for whom there are no contraindications	10 points	40–80%

Coronary heart disease: 📖 p.245

Hypertension: 📖 p.253

Diabetes: 📖 p.255

Investigations

ECG: 80–90% of patients with heart failure have some or all of the following ECG changes:
- Q-waves
- ST/T-wave changes
- Left ventricular hypertrophy
- Various arrhythmias
- Conduction disturbances.

Natriuretic peptides: These exert a wide range of effects on the heart, kidney and CNS. The most useful measurement is of brain natriuretic peptide (BNP) which is also released from the heart. Natriuretic peptides act as a physiological antagonist to the effects of angiotensin II and are increasingly being used as diagnostic markers of heart failure.

Echo: 📖 p.54. Confirms diagnosis and gives an objective measure of left ventricular function[£].

Management: 📖 p.82.

Prognosis: Progressive deterioration to death. ~½ die suddenly probably due to arrhythmias. *Mortality:*
- Mild/moderate heart failure – 20–30% 1y. mortality
- Severe heart failure – >50% 1y. mortality.

A number of factors correlate with the prognosis:
- Clinical – the worse the patient's symptoms, the worse the prognosis
- Haemodynamics – the lower the cardiac index, stroke volume and ejection fraction, the worse the prognosis
- Biochemical – certain endocrine markers and hyponatraemia are associated with a poorer prognosis
- Arrhythmias – frequent ventricular ectopics or ventricular tachycardia on ambulatory ECG indicate a poorer prognosis.

Further information

NICE Chronic heart failure (2003) 🖥 www.nice.org.uk
Davis, R. et al. *ABC of heart failure* (2006) BMJ Books. ISBN: 0727916440

Advice for patients: Patient experiences of chronic heart failure

Breathlessness

'When I started getting very alarmingly puffy, and especially alarming was getting breathless lying down in bed, I thought well this is not right, this is something wrong … I went down to the local doctor … and she decided to send me for a scan in the [name of hospital] hospital.'

'Shortness of breath, you know, wanting to do things more or less out of the ordinary, such as gardening, you know. Out of my ordinary scope, of course, I can't, because shortness of breath steps in and you can feel your heart sometimes, you know? You can feel it's there, it starts to … you can feel the beat. And when I start to feel the beat then I know it's time to slow down.'

'If I'm lying flat then often I'll wake up probably breathless but maybe with a coughing attack. Coughing is a real problem for me when I'm flat. And I also wake up early in the morning, when I wake up at 4 o'clock, 5 o'clock, 6 o'clock, but I'll often go off to sleep again for a bit, but I'm always up by 7. Just to go to bed and have an uninterrupted night's sleep and wake up at 8 o'clock would be delicious, but it isn't happening, and we're nearly two years in now, so I don't think it's going to come back.'

Work tolerance

'I can do half as much as I used to. I can't do hard work now, or heavy work, no. I can do light work, and I could go all day, but I couldn't do hard work, no.'

Tiredness

'It's not a "tired" tired where you want to go to bed and sleep, it's a weary tired, as if everything is an effort. It's a tired where you don't want to go to bed and sleep, you just want to, I don't know, it's like a weary tired, that's the only way I can describe it really. I can't say it's a "go to sleep" tired. I don't really know, it's just an "I must sit down" tired, "I just can't take another step" tired.'

Information for patients and their carers

British Heart Foundation ☎ 0845 0708 070 🖥 www.bhf.org.uk
DIPEx Database of personal and health experiences: heart failure 🖥 www.dipex.org

Management of chronic heart failure

🚹 Always look for the underlying cause and treat wherever possible. Review the basis for historical diagnoses and arrange echo to confirm diagnosis is in doubt.

Non-drug measures

- *Educate* – about the disease, current/expected symptoms and need for treatment. Discuss prognosis. Support with written information.
- *Discuss ways to make life easier* e.g. benefits, mobility aids, blue disability parking badge. Consider referral to social services for assessment for services such as home care.
- *Diet* – ensure adequate calories, ↓ salt, ↓ weight if obese, restrict alcohol.
- *Lifestyle measures* – smoking cessation[£] (📖 p.188), regular exercise.
- *Restrict fluid intake* – if severe heart failure.
- *Vaccination* – influenza and pneumococcal vaccination[£].
- *Assess for depression* – common amongst patients with heart failure.

Drug treatment: Table 3.4, 📖 p.84.
Aims to
- Improve symptoms – diuretics, digoxin and ACE inhibitors[£] *and*
- Improve survival – ACE inhibitors[£], β-blockers, oral nitrates + hydralazine, spironolactone.

Algorithm for drug treatment of heart failure: Figure 3.3.

Monitoring: Review every 6mo. or more often as required. Check:
- *Clinical state* – functional capacity (Table 3.3, 📖 p.79), fluid status, cardiac rhythm, cognitive and nutritional status, mood
- *Medication* – ensure drug record is up to date, review compliance and side-effects, change drugs if clinical circumstances/best practice alter
- *Blood* – U&E and creatinine.

Referral to general medicine, cardiology or elderly care

- Heart failure unable to be managed at home – E
- Severe heart failure – U/S
- Heart failure not controlled by medication – U/S/R
- Angina, AF or other symptomatic arrhythmias – U/S/R
- If diagnosis is in doubt – S/R
- To initiate an ACE inhibitor or β-blocker (see Table 3.4 📖 p.84) – S/R
- Heart failure due to valve disease or diastolic dysfunction – R
- Co-morbidity that may impact on heart failure (COPD, renal dysfunction, anaemia, thyroid disease, peripheral vascular disease, urinary frequency, gout) – R
- Women with heart failure planning pregnancy – R

E = Emergency admission; U = Urgent; S = Soon; R = Routine

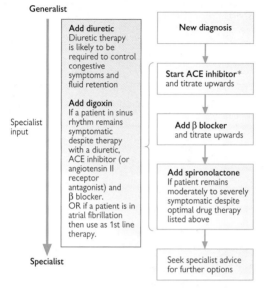

Figure 3.3 NICE algorithm for pharmacological treatment of symptomatic heart failure due to left ventricular systolic dysfunction

Generalist

Add diuretic
Diuretic therapy is likely to be required to control congestive symptoms and fluid retention

Add digoxin
If a patient in sinus rhythm remains symptomatic despite therapy with a diuretic, ACE inhibitor (or angiotensin II receptor antagonist) and β blocker.
OR if a patient is in atrial fibrillation then use as 1st line therapy.

Specialist input

Specialist

New diagnosis

Start ACE inhibitor*
and titrate upwards

Add β blocker
and titrate upwards

Add spironolactone
If patient remains moderately to severely symptomatic despite optimal drug therapy listed above

Seek specialist advice for further options

* If ACE inhibitor is not tolerated (e.g. due to severe cough) consider an angiotensin II receptor antagonist

Further information

NICE Chronic heart failure (2003) 🖥 www.nice.org.uk
SIGN Management of chronic heart failure (2007) 🖥 www.sign.ac.uk

Advice for patients: Patient information

British Heart Foundation ☎ 0845 0708 070 🖥 www.bhf.org.uk

Table 3.4 Drugs used in the treatment of chronic heart failure

Drug class	Treatment notes
Diuretics BNF 2.2	*Loop diuretics* e.g. furosemide or *thiazides* e.g. bendroflume-thiazide. Use the minimum effective dose to control congestive symptoms and fluid retention (e.g. furosemide 20mg od). Monitor for ↓ K$^+$ – co-treat with amiloride, ACE inhibitor or K$^+$ supplement as necessary.
ACE inhibitors BNF 2.5.5.1 ⬤ Check U&E and Cr before starting, at first follow-up and after each ↑ dose ⚠ *Do not use:* If renovascular disease, in pregnancy, if the patient has HOCM or if significant valve disease	Improve symptoms,↑ exercise capacity, ↓ progression of disease , ↓ hospital admissions and ↑ survival in symptomatic and asymptomatic patients. Start at low dose (e.g. ramipril 1.25mg od) and titrate upwards. Refer for specialist initiation if: • Age ≥70y • Severe or unstable heart failure • Hypovolaemia • Hypotension – systolic BP <90mmHg • Hyponatraemia (Na$^+$ <130mmol/l) • Renal impairment (creatinine >150μmol/l) • Receiving multiple or high-dose diuretic therapy (e.g. >80mg furosemide/d.) or high-dose vasodilator therapy If ACE inhibitors are not tolerated consider an angiotensin receptor blocker (ARB).
β-blockers BNF 2.4 ⬤ Refer for specialist initiation if any contraindication, elderly or severe heart failure	Start a β-blocker licensed for heart failure (e.g. bisoprolol 1.25mg mane) after diuretic and ACE inhibitor in all those with left ventricular dysfunction regardless of whether symptoms persist. Use in a 'start low, go slow' approach with assessment of pulse, BP and clinical status after each titration upwards, over a matter of a few months.
Digoxin BNF 2.1.1	Use when symptoms persist despite ACE inhibitor, β-blocker and diuretics, and for patients with AF + heart failure. 2 effects – antiarrhythmic and +ve inotrope. Improves symptoms, exercise tolerance and → ↓ admissions to hospital. No improvement in overall survival.
Other drugs to consider depending on co-existent conditions	*Anticoagulation* – patients with heart failure and AF, past history of thromboembolism, left ventricular aneurysm or intrathoracic thrombus – 📖 p.158. *Aspirin* – 75–150mg od if heart failure + atherosclerotic arterial disease (including CHD). *Statins* – only if other indications – 📖 p.186. *Amlodipine* – can be used for treatment of angina and ↑ BP in patients with heart failure. ⬤ *Avoid* verapamil, diltiazem or short-acting dihydropyridine agents.
Drugs initiated under specialist supervision only	*Amiodarone* – all patients require clinical review, LFTs and TFTs every 6mo. (📖 p.95) *Spironolactone* – ↑ survival if severe heart failure. Refer if moderate or severe symptoms after MI and/or despite optimal therapy. Dose 12.5–50mg od – monitor for ↑ K$^+$ and ↓ renal function. If ↑ K$^+$, ½ the dose and recheck. *Isosorbide/hydralazine combination.* *Inotropic agents.*

GMS contract			
HF 1	The practice can produce a register of patients with heart failure	4 points	
HF 2	% of patients with a diagnosis of heart failure (diagnosed after 01.04.2006) which has been confirmed by an echocardiogram or by specialist assessment	6 points	40–90%
HF 3	% of patients with a current diagnosis of heart failure due to left ventricular dysfunction who are currently treated with an ACE inhibitor or Angiotensin Receptor Blocker, who can tolerate therapy and for whom there is no contraindications	10 points	40–80%

Coronary heart disease: 📖 p.245
Hypertension: 📖 p.253
Diabetes: 📖 p.255

GP Notes: Frequently asked questions about digoxin

How do I start digoxin?
In the community give 125–250mcgm digoxin bd po for 1wk. then 125mcgm od. ↓ dose for patients who are elderly, have taken digoxin in the previous 2wk., are taking amiodarone or verapamil, or have renal failure.

What is the maintenance dose of digoxin?
Maintenance dose is 62.5–500mcgm/d. po. Higher doses may be divided to avoid nausea. Adjust dose according to response, toxicity and serum levels. Maintenance dose can usually be determined by ventricular rate at rest – do not allow rate to fall to <60bpm.

Do I need to monitor digoxin levels?
Regular monitoring is not necessary unless problems occur – use to assess whether adverse symptoms are due to toxicity (though plasma concentration alone does not reliably indicate toxicity – the likelihood of toxicity ↑ as the level ↑).

Measure plasma digoxin level >6h. after the last dose. Normal range is 1.2–1.9ng/ml. Toxicity is likely if >2.5ng/ml

Is there anything else I should check?
Low K^+ and renal failure predispose to toxicity. Monitor at least annually (every 6mo. if the patient is taking a diuretic). For patients taking diuretics, use K^+ sparing diuretics or K^+ supplements routinely.

What are the symptoms of toxicity?
Symtoms include: anorexia, nausea, vomiting, abdominal pain, diarrhoea, headache, confusion, visual symptoms and arrhythmias (e.g. heart block, VT).

Stop until symptoms resolve then restart at lower dose. If severe digoxin toxicity, deliberate or inadvertent overdose, or arrhythmia – admit.

Pulmonary hypertension and cor pulmonale

Normal pulmonary arterial pressure is $<\frac{1}{5}$ of that in the systemic circulation. Pulmonary hypertension occurs by one of 3 mechanisms:

- High pulmonary blood flow (e.g. left → right shunt)
- ↑ pulmonary vascular resistance
- Chronic pulmonary venous hypertension.

Causes of pulmonary hypertension

- **Lung disease:** Asthma; bronchiectasis; pulmonary fibrosis
- **Cardiac disease:** Mitral stenosis; congenital heart disease; severe LVF
- **Hypoventilation:** Sleep apnoea; enlarged adenoids in children; CVA
- **Pulmonary vascular disease:** PE; sickle-cell disease
- **Neuromuscular disease:** MND; polio; myaesthenia gravis
- **Thoracic cage abnormalities:** Kyphosis; scoliosis

Consequences of pulmonary hypertension

- With time, ↑ pressure in the pulmonary vascular tree results in permanent damage to smaller pulmonary vessels and pulmonary hypertension becomes irreversible – even if the cause is removed.
- If a shunt is present, when pulmonary pressure > systemic pressure the shunt reverses and the patient becomes cyanotic (Eisenmenger's syndrome).

Diagnosis: Underdiagnosed – delay between onset of symptoms and diagnosis is ~2y.

Presentation: CCF ± infective bronchitis, chest pain, breathlessness lethargy and fatigue, haemoptysis, syncope, nausea.

Examination: Check for cyanosis, peripheral oedema, ↑ JVP, 4th heart sound, diastolic murmur from pulmonary regurgitation, hepatomegaly ± ascites, crepitations at lung bases ± pleural effusion.

Investigations

- **CXR** – cardiomegaly + enlargement of proximal pulmonary arteries.
- **ECG** – right axis deviation, tall peaked P waves and dominant R wave in right precordial leads *or* RBBB.

Management: Refer to cardiologist or chest physician. Doppler echo is used to assess ventricular function and pulmonary arterial pressure. In the UK, ongoing care is now organized into designated multidisciplinary pulmonary hypertension units.

Treatment

- Remove the underlying cause if possible.
- Oxygen therapy for symptomatic relief.
- Epoprostenol analogues have now become the mainstay of treatment. They ↑ exercise tolerance and survival. Bosentan is also used.
- Vasodilation with calcium-channel blockers (in the 10–15% of patients who are responsive) can dramatically improve prognosis.
- Treat left ventricular failure with ACE inhibitors, β-blockers & diuretics.
- Anticoagulation.

Prognosis: If the cause is irreversible, a steady decline towards cor pulmonale and death is the likely outcome and heart–lung transplantation the only option. However, newer drugs are improving prognosis.

Pulmonary hypertension and pregnancy: Risk of death is high in conditions where pulmonary blood flow cannot be ↑ e.g. Eisenmenger's syndrome (maternal mortality 30–50%); primary pulmonary hypertension (mortality 40–50%).

Management: Specialist obstetric care is required for all patients with a pre-existing cardiac condition. Where possible refer pre-conception to a cardiologist for discussion of risks. Antibiotic prophylaxis is necessary for women with structural cardiac disease for delivery – 📖 p.100.

Cor pulmonale: Right heart failure as a result of chronic hypoxia causing chronic pulmonary hypertension. Due to diseases of the lung, its vessels or the thoracic cage.

Further information
British Heart Foundation Factfile *Pulmonary hypertension* (01/2003)
🖥 www.bhf.org.uk

Tachycardia and palpitations

Heart rate >100bpm. Palpitations are the sensation of rapid, irregular or forceful heartbeats. Common and may be an incidental finding. History and examination can exclude significant problems in most patients.

History: Ask about:
- *Palpitations* – duration, frequency and pattern, rhythm (ask the patient to tap it out if not present when seen)
- *Precipitating/relieving factors*
- *Associated symptoms* – chest pain, collapse or funny turns, sweating, breathlessness or hyperventilation
- *Past history* e.g. previous episodes, heart disease, thyroid disease
- *Lifestyle* – drug history, caffeine/alcohol intake, smoking
- *Occupation* – arrhythmias may affect driving (📖 p.222) and/or work.

> ⚠ **Red flag symptoms**
> - Pre-existing cardiovascular disease
> - FH of syncope, arrhythmia or sudden death
> - Arrhythmia associated with falls and/or syncope

Examination
- *General examination* – for anaemia, thyrotoxicosis, anxiety, other systemic disease
- *Cardiovascular examination* – heart size, pulse rate and rhythm, JVP, BP, heart sounds and murmurs, evidence of left ventricular failure

Investigations
First-line: Resting ECG is all that is needed for many patients.

Further investigations: Consider if ECG is abnormal or other concerning features:
- Ambulatory ECG or cardiac memo
- Echo if <50y. or murmur/left ventricular failure detected
- Exercise tolerance test if exercise related
- *Blood:* TFTs, FBC, ESR, U&E, fasting blood glucose, Ca^{2+}, albumin.

> **Ventricular tachycardia (VT):** Broad (>3 small squares) QRS complexes at a rate of >100bpm on ECG (Figure 3.4).
>
> **Management**
> - Admit as blue-light emergency.
> - Meanwhile give O_2 if available ± 100mg IV lidocaine.
> - If no pulse treat as VF cardiac arrest (📖 p.10).
>
> **Recurrent VT:** May require surgery, insertion of a pacemaker or implantable cardioverter defibrillator.

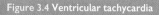

Figure 3.4 Ventricular tachycardia

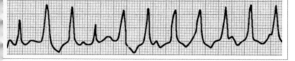

Figure 3.5 Ventricular fibrillation

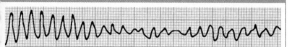

GP Notes: NSF for coronary heart disease recommendations

- *Referral to a heart rhythm expert:* All 1st degree relatives of sudden cardiac death patients who died age <40y.
- *Referral to a paediatric cardiologist:* Any child with:
  - Recurrent loss of consciousness
  - Collapse on exertion
  - Atypical seizure and normal EEG
  - Documented arrhythmia

Further Information

National Service Framework for coronary heart disease (2005)
⌨ www.dh.gov.uk

Ventricular ectopic beats: Additional broad QRS complexes, without P waves, superimposed on regular sinus rhythm (Figure 3.6). Common and usually of no clinical significance. Rarely may be the presenting feature of viral myocarditis. *Management:*

- *Frequent ectopics (>100/h.) on ECG:* Refer urgently to cardiology
- *R on T phenomenon on ECG:* Rarely ectopics can cause ventricular fibrillation, particularly if coinciding with the T wave of a preceding beat ('R on T phenomenon' – Figure 3.7). If occurs >10x/min. – admit.
- *After MI:* Ventricular extrasystoles after MI are associated with ↑ mortality. Refer to cardiology.
- *No sinister features on ECG:* Explain the benign nature of the condition. Advise avoidance of caffeine, alcohol, smoking and fatigue. β-blockers can be helpful for patients unable to tolerate ectopics despite reassurance.

Sinus tachycardia: Consider infection, pain, MI, shock, exercise, emotion (including anxiety), heart failure, thyrotoxicosis, drugs.

Paroxysmal supraventricular tachycardia (SVT): Narrow QRS complex tachycardia with a regular rate >100bpm on ECG (Figure 3.8).

Management

If seen during an attack
- Get an ECG if possible.
- Try carotid sinus massage (unless elderly, IHD, digoxin toxic, carotid bruit, history of TIAs), the Valsalva manoeuvre and/or ice on the face (especially effective for children).
- Admit as an emergency if the attack continues.
- If the attack stops, refer to cardiology for advice on further management, enclosing a copy of the ECG trace during an attack if available.

If diagnosed from history or ambulatory ECG trace: Refer to cardiology for confirmation of diagnosis and initiation of treatment – urgent referral if chest pain, dizziness or breathlessness during attacks. Enclose the ECG trace during an attack if available.

Treatment options are: sotalol, verapamil or amiodarone (📖 p.95).

Advice: Advise patients to avoid caffeine, alcohol and smoking.

Wolff-Parkinson-White (WPW) syndrome: A congenital accessory conduction pathway is present between atrium and ventricle (bundle of Kent). *Clinical features:*
- Predisposes to SVT and AF.
- *ECG:* short P–R interval followed by slurred upstroke ('delta wave') into the QRS complex – Figure 3.9.
- *Management:* Refer to cardiology. Treatment is with anti-arrhythmics (SVT – verapamil; AF – amiodarone or DC shock) ± ablation of the accessory pathway.

Atrial fibrillation/flutter: 📖 p.92.

No tachycardia and no ECG abnormalities: Reassure. Explore the possibility of an anxiety disorder.

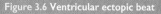

Figure 3.6 Ventricular ectopic beat

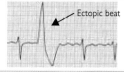

Ectopic beat

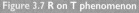

Figure 3.7 R on T phenomenon

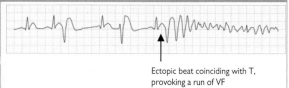

Ectopic beat coinciding with T,
provoking a run of VF

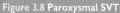

Figure 3.8 Paroxysmal SVT

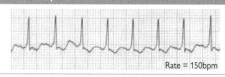

Rate = 150bpm

Figure 3.9 Wolff-Parkinson-White syndrome

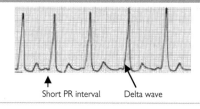

Short PR interval   Delta wave

Further information

Morris, F. et al. *ABC of clinical electrocardiography* (2002) BMJ Books.
ISBN: 0727915363
British Heart Foundation Factfile *Palpitations: their significance and
investigation* (04/2004) 🖳 www.bhf.org.uk
NEJM Huikuri et al. *Sudden death due to cardiac arrhythmias* (2001) **345**
pp. 1473–1482
NICE Implantable cardioverter defibrillators, (ICDs) for the treatment
of arrhythmias – a review of guidance **no.11** (2006).
🖳 www.nice.org.uk

Figure 3.7 is reproduced from Morris F, Edhouse J, Brady W, and Camm J, (2002), The *ABC of
Clinical Electrocardiography*, with permission from Blackwell BMJ Books.

Atrial fibrillation (AF)^G

A common disturbance of cardiac rhythm which may be episodic (*paroxysmal*) or chronic. Characterized by rapid irregularly irregular narrow QRS complex tachycardia with absence of P waves. Affects <1% <60y., but >8% aged over 80y. Associated with 5x ↑ risk of stroke (📖 p.122).

Causes
- No cause (isolated AF) ~12%
- Coronary heart disease
- Valvular heart disease (especially mitral valve disease)
- ↑ BP (especially if left ventricular hypertrophy)
- Cardiomyopathy

Acute AF: May be precipitated by acute infection, high alcohol intake, surgery, electrocution, MI, pericarditis, PE or hyperthyroidism.

Symptoms: Often asymptomatic but may cause palpitations, chest pain, stroke/TIA, dyspnoea, fatigue, light-headedness and/or syncope.

Examination
- *General examination:* Check for anaemia, thyrotoxicosis, anxiety, and other systemic disease.
- *Cardiovascular examination:* Check heart size, pulse rate and rhythm (apex rate > radial pulse rate when a patient is in AF), JVP, BP, heart sounds and murmurs, and for evidence of left ventricular failure.

Investigations
- Resting ECG (Figure 3.10)
- CXR
- *Blood:* TFTs, FBC, U&E

Further investigations
- Ambulatory ECG – if suspected asymptomatic episodes of paroxysmal AF or symptomatic episodes <24h. apart
- Cardiac memo – if symptomatic episodes of paroxysmal AF >24h apart
- Echo – if <50y. or murmur/left ventricular failure detected
- Exercise tolerance test – if exercise related.

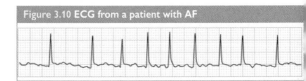

Figure 3.10 **ECG from a patient with AF**

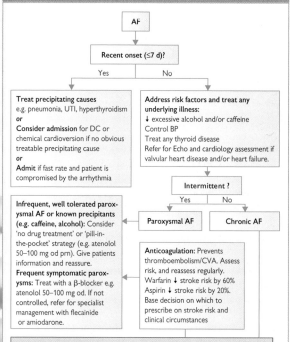

Figure 3.11 Management of AF in primary care

AF

Recent onset (≤7 d)?

Yes — No

Treat precipitating causes
e.g. pneumonia, UTI, hyperthyroidism
or
Consider admission for DC or chemical cardioversion if no obvious treatable precipitating cause
or
Admit if fast rate and patient is compromised by the arrhythmia

Address risk factors and treat any underlying illness:
↓ excessive alcohol and/or caffeine
Control BP
Treat any thyroid disease
Refer for Echo and cardiology assessment if valvular heart disease and/or heart failure.

Intermittent ?

Yes — No

Paroxysmal AF — Chronic AF

Infrequent, well tolerated paroxysmal AF or known precipitants (e.g. caffeine, alcohol): Consider 'no drug treatment' or 'pill-in-the-pocket' strategy (e.g. atenolol 50–100 mg od prn). Give patients information and reassure.
Frequent symptomatic paroxysms: Treat with a β-blocker e.g. atenolol 50–100 mg od. If not controlled, refer for specialist management with flecainide or amiodarone.

Anticoagulation: Prevents thromboembolism/CVA. Assess risk, and reassess regularly.
Warfarin ↓ stroke risk by 60%
Aspirin ↓ stroke risk by 20%.
Base decision on which to prescribe on stroke risk and clinical circumstances

2 treatment approaches:
Rhythm-control: Consider referral/ admission for DC or chemical cardioversion to restore sinus rhythm if:
—Symptomatic or CCF   —Age ≤65 y
—First presentation with lone AF   —AF 2° to a treated/corrected precipitant
❶ After treatment, medication (e.g. β-blocker) may be needed to maintain sinus rhythm.
Rate control: Consider controlling ventricular rate with a β-blocker (e.g. atenolol 50–100 mg od) or rate limiting calcium antagonist (e.g. verapamil 40–120 mg tds) if:
—Age >65 y   —Long duration of AF (>12 mo)
—Coronary artery disease   —No CCF
—Structural heart disease that makes AF likely, e.g. mitral stenosis, large left atrium
—History of multiple failed attempts at cardioversion/relapses
—Contraindications to anticoagulation
—Ongoing but reversible cause of AF, e.g. thyrotoxicosis.
Aim for a ventricular rate of 60–80 bpm at rest and 90–115 bpm during moderate exercise. If ineffective during normal activities combine a β-blocker with digoxin; if ineffective during exercise combine a rate limiting calcium antagonist with digoxin
If still ineffective/poorly tolerated—refer for consideration of other anti-arrhythmic agents e.g. sotalol, propafenone, flecainide, or amiodarone
❶ Consider digoxin as monotherapy for predominantly sedentary patients

93

Management: Figure 3.11 📖 p.93. Aims to:
- Relieve symptoms e.g. palpitations, fatigue, dyspnoea
- Prevent thromboembolism and ↓ risk of stroke *and*
- Maintain cardiac function

'Pill-in-the-pocket' approach to paroxysmal AF: Consider offering self-medication with a β-blocker (e.g. atenolol 50–100mg od) to use as needed if infrequent symptomatic paroxysms and:
- No history of left ventricular dysfunction, valvular or ischaemic heart disease
- Systolic BP >100mgHg and resting heart rate >70bpm
- Able to understand when and how to take the medication

Anticoagulation around cardioversion
- If AF was <48h, duration before successful cardioversion – no anticoagulation required
- If routine elective cardioversion – anticoagulation with warfarin for 3wk. prior to the procedure (aim INR 2–3)
- Following cardioversion (except if AF of <48h, duration before cardioversion) – anticoagulation with warfarin for at least 4wk. (aim INR 2–3). Consider long-term anticoagulation to prevent stroke (📖 p.126) or if high risk of recurrence–previous failed attempts/ recurrences, prolonged AF (>12 mo.), or structural heart disease (mitral valve disease, left ventricular dysfunction, enlarged left atrium).

Use of digoxin: 📖 p.85

Referral to cardiology, general medicine or elderly care
- Fast rate and patient compromised by arrhythmia (chest pain, ↓ BP or more than mild heart failure) – E
- Candidate for DC or chemical cardioversion – E/U
- Uncertainty about diagnosis or treatment – S/R
- Symptoms are uncontrolled by standard treatment – S/R
- Paroxysmal AF for consideration of sotalol or other anti-arrythmic drugs when standard β-blockers have failed – S/R

E = Emergency admission; U = Urgent; S = Soon; R = Routine

Risk of stroke associated with AF: 📖 p.127

Atrial flutter: ECG shows regular saw-tooth baseline at rate of 300bpm with a narrow QRS complex tachycardia superimposed at a rate of 150bpm or 100bpm. Manage in the same way as AF (though specialist drug treatment may differ).

Further information
NICE Atrial fibrillation: the management of atrial fibrillation (2006) 🖥 www.nice.org.uk

GMS contract			
AF 1	The practice can produce a register of patients with atrial fibrillation	5 points	
AF 2	% of patients with atrial fibrillation diagnosed from 01.04.2006 with ECG or specialist confirmed diagnosis	up to 10 points	40–90%
AF 3	% of patients with atrial fibrillation who are currently treated with anti-coagulant drug therapy or an anti-platelet therapy	up to 15 points	40–90%

GP Notes: Frequently asked questions about use of amiodarone

BNF 2.3.2

What is amiodarone?
Amiodarone is an anti-arrhythmic agent which causes very little myocardial depression. It is used for the treatment of arrhythmias (e.g. SVT, AF/atrial flutter, VT, VF), particularly when other drugs have failed.

How do I start amiodarone?
⚠ *Always start in hospital or under specialist supervision.*

- Check baseline CXR, liver function tests and TFTs.
- Very long ½ life, so requires a loading dose and plasma concentration may take weeks to reach steady state. In the community – start with 200mg tds for 1wk. followed by 200mg bd for 1wk. then 200mg od or the minimum dose needed to control the arrhythmia.
- Divide higher doses to avoid nausea.
- Interactions with other drugs may take some time to have effect due to the long ½ life of amiodarone.

What are the contraindications of amiodarone?
Contraindications include: iodine sensitivity, bradycardia/heart block, pregnancy/breast feeding.

What monitoring is needed?
Monitor thyroid function tests and liver function tests every 6mo.

What are the side-effects of amiodarone treatment?
Side-effects include:

- *Microcorneal deposits* (reverse on withdrawal) – common – rarely ↓ vision – but may cause dazzle when driving at night
- *Phototoxic reactions* – advise to stay out of the sun, cover up and wear broad-spectrum sunscreen
- *Hypo/hyperthyroidism*
- *Peripheral neuropathy/myopathy* – usually reversible
- *Bradycardia/conduction disturbances*
- *Liver abnormalities*
- *Pulmonary fibrosis.*

Bradycardia

Heart rate <60bpm.

Presentation: Often an incidental finding but may present with faints or blackouts, drop attacks, dizziness, breathlessness or lack of energy.

Examination: Slow pulse rate; normal or low BP ± evidence of 2° heart failure. There may also be symptoms/signs of associated disease.

Investigations

- *ECG:* See opposite; ambulatory ECG may help with diagnosis of intermittent bradycardia (e.g. sick sinus syndrome).
- *Blood:* TFTs, FBC, ESR, U&E, LFTs, digoxin levels (if taking digoxin).

Sinus bradycardia: Constant bradycardia. P waves present and P–R interval <0.2sec. (1 large square) – Figure 3.12. *Causes:*

- Physiological e.g. athletes
- Vasovagal attack
- Drugs e.g. β-blockers, digoxin
- Inferior MI
- Sick sinus syndrome
- Hypothyroidism
- Hypothermia
- ↑ ICP
- Jaundice

Management: Admit acutely if symptomatic. Refer for cardiology opinion if asymptomatic but HR <40bpm despite treatment of reversible causes.

AV node block (heart block): *Causes:*

- IHD
- Drugs (digoxin, verapamil)
- Myocarditis
- Cardiomyopathy
- Fibrosis
- Lyme disease (rare)

Types of heart block

1st degree block – fixed P–R interval >200ms (1 large square) – Figure 3.13

2nd degree block

- *Mobitz type I* (Wenckebach) – progressively lengthening P–R interval followed by a dropped beat – Figure 3.14
- *Mobitz type II* – constant P–R interval with regular dropped beats (e.g. 2:1 – every 2nd beat is dropped – consider drug toxicity) – Figure 3.14.

3rd degree block *(complete heart block)* P–P intervals are constant and R–R intervals are constant but not related to each other – Figure 3.15

Management: Untreated 2nd and 3rd degree heart block have a mortality of ≈35%. Refer all patients to cardiology even if asymptomatic. If symptomatic (↓BP <90mmHg systolic, left ventricular failure, heart rate <40bpm) admit as an emergency – give IV atropine and O₂ (if available) whilst awaiting admission.

Stokes-Adams attacks: Cardiac arrest due to AV block. Results in sudden loss of consciousness ± some limb twitching due to cerebral anoxia. The patient becomes pale and pulseless but respiration continues. Attacks usually lasts ~30sec. though occasionally are fatal. On recovery the patient becomes flushed. Refer to cardiology if suspected.

Figure 3.12 Sinus bradycardia

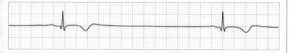

Figure 3.13 1ˢᵗ degree heart block

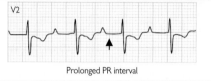

V2

Prolonged PR interval

Figure 3.14 2ⁿᵈ degree heart block

Mobitz type I

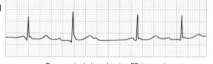

Progressively lengthening PR interval

Mobitz type II

Dropped beat

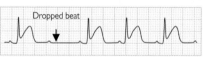

Constant PR interval – regular dropped beats

Figure 3.15 3ʳᵈ degree (complete) heart block

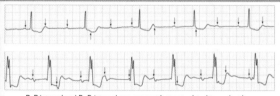

P–P interval and R–R interval are constant but not related to each other
(P waves are marked)

Figures 3.13, 3.14 and 3.15 are reproduced from Morris F, Edhouse J, Brady W, and Camm J, (2002), The *ABC of Clinical Electrocardiography*, with permission from Blackwell BMJ Books.

Sick sinus syndrome: Due to sinus node dysfunction causing brady-cardia ± asystole, sinoatrial block (complete heart block), AF or SVT alternating with bradycardia (tachy/brady syndrome). Common amongst elderly patients. If symptomatic, heart rate <40bpm or pauses >3s. on ECG (Figure 3.16), refer to cardiology for pacemaker insertion.

Pacemakers: Electrically stimulate the heart to beat. *Indications:*
- Symptomatic bradycardia
- 2nd or 3rd degree heart block
- Temporary suppression of resistant tachycardia.

Insertion: Pacemaker box is attached under the skin of the chest – usually medial to the left axilla under local anaesthetic. Wires are fed via the great veins of the chest to the heart under X-ray and/or US guidance.

Types: Classified according to:
- Chamber paced – atrium, ventricle or both ('dual')
- Chamber sensed – atrium, ventricle or both ('dual')
- Mode of response to sensing – inhibited output, triggered, inhibited and triggered ('dual').

Therefore, a VVI pacemaker paces the ventricle ('V'), and senses the ventricle ('V'). In inhibited mode ('I'), if the ventricle beats spontane-ously the pacemaker will not fire.

ECG changes with a pacemaker: If the pacemaker is in operation a pacing 'spike' (vertical line) is seen on ECG (Figure 3.17).

ⓘ In devices pacing on demand, a spike will not be seen if the natural rate is in excess of the rate set on the pacemaker.

Lifespan: Pacemakers last 7–15y. Regular checks are made by pace-maker clinics to ensure the pacemaker remains operational. Repro-gramming through the skin is possible. Batteries can be changed via a small surgical procedure under local anaesthetic.

Driving with a pacemaker: Inform DVLA and insurance company (📖 p.220). Stop driving for 1mo. after insertion.

⚠ After death, pacemakers must be removed before cremation can take place. A fee is payable.

Further information

Morris, F. et al. *ABC of electrocardiology* (2002) BMJ Books. ISBN 0727915363

NEJM Mangrum & DiMarco *The evaluation and management of bradycardia* (2000) **342:** pp. 703–709

Figure 3.16 Pause of >3sec. in a patient with sick sinus syndrome

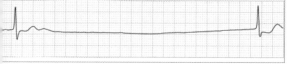

Figure 3.17 ECG of a patient with a ventricular pacemaker

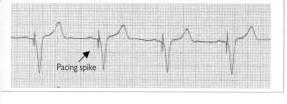

Pacing spike

Infective endocarditis

⚠ New murmur + fever = endocarditis until proven otherwise.

Infective endocarditis occurs when there is infection of a heart valve. The valve may be normal (50% – may be associated with IV drug abuse), rheumatic, degenerative, congenitally abnormal or prosthetic (Table 3.5). Uncommon but consequences may be disastrous and often detected late.

Causes
- *Common organisms:* Strep. viridans (35–50%); Staph. aureus (20%).
- *Non-bacterial causes:* SLE, malignancy.

Presentation: May be acute (acute heart failure) or subacute (course worsening over days/weeks). *Symptoms/signs:*
- *Infective* – fever, weight ↓, night sweats, malaise, lethargy, clubbing, splenomegaly, anaemia, mycotic aneurysms
- *Heart murmurs ± heart failure*
- *Embolic* – stroke, lung abscesses (right heart endocarditis)
- *Vasculitic* – Figure 2.3, 📖 p.25 – microscopic haematuria, splinter haemorrhages, Osler's nodes (painful lesions on finger pulps), Janeway lesions (palmar macules), Roth's spots (retinal vasculitis), conjunctival petechiae, renal failure.

Management: Have a high index of suspicion for patients at ↑ risk i.e. with valve lesions or prosthetic valves. Admit as an emergency if suspected. Avoid starting antibiotics prior to admission as this might cause delay in diagnosis by rendering the blood cultures sterile. Hospital treatment is with prolonged IV broad-spectrum antibiotics (≥2wk.).

Prognosis: 20–25% of those admitted with a diagnosis of infective endocarditis die; 80% have major complications during admission e.g. heart failure. Valve replacement may be required – especially if endocarditis is on a prosthetic valve.

Table 3.5 Risk of developing infective endocarditis

Risk	Condition	Antibiotic prophylaxis
High	Prosthetic heart valve Past history of infective endocarditis Complex cyanotic congenital heart disease	Required
Moderate	Mitral valve prolapse[*] Valvular dysfunction (e.g. following rheumatic heart disease) Ventricular septal defects Primum atrial septal defects HOCM Past history of rheumatic fever	Required
Low	Murmurs not due to valve disease e.g. flow murmurs in pregnancy	Not required

[*] If audible mitral regurgitation or Echo shows regurgitation or thickened (myxomatous) mitral valve leaflets.

Prevention: Those at high/moderate risk of infective endocarditis (Table 3.5) should take prophylactic antibiotics prior to any procedure that might cause a transient bacteraemia (Tables 3.6 & 3.7). Good dental hygiene is also important, including regular dentist check-ups.

Table 3.6 Procedures requiring antibiotic prophylaxis

Procedures requiring prophylaxis		Procedures not requiring prophylaxis
High & moderate-risk patients	**High-risk patients only**	
Dental procedures which can → gum bleeding (i.e. virtually all dental procedures)	All endoscopic procedures including proctoscopy and sigmoidoscopy	Routine phlebotomy
		Cervical smear
	Normal obstetric delivery	Insertion of IV cannula (though should be changed frequently)
Surgery (excluding skin surgery) – warn consultant in referral letter	Insertion of IUCD	
Lower GI or GU endoscopy	Insertion of a urethral catheter in a patient with infected urine (ensure infecting organism is sensitive to prophylactic antibiotics)	

⚠ If in doubt ask advice from the cardiologist in charge of the patient's care or a specialist in infectious diseases.

Table 3.7 Antibiotic regimes for use in primary care BNF 5.1

Patients	Antibiotics
• All patients *except* • those with a past history of endocarditis • those who are penicillin-allergic • those who have had >1 dose of penicillin in the previous month	Amoxicillin 3g po 1h. before the procedure (child <5y. – ¼ adult dose; child 5–10y. – ½ adult dose)
Patients allergic to penicillin *or* Patients who have received >1 dose of penicillin in the previous month	Clindamycin 600mg po 1h. before the procedure (child <5y. – ¼ adult dose; child 5–10y. – ½ adult dose)
Patients with a past history of endocarditis	The procedure should be carried out in hospital with IV gentamicin 120mg prior to the procedure then amoxicillin 500mg 6h. after the procedure

101

Further information

British Heart Foundation Factfiles *Infective endocarditis* (12/2003 & 1/2004) 🖳 www.bhf.org.uk

Rheumatic fever and myocarditis

There has been a dramatic ↓ in incidence of rheumatic fever in industrialized countries since the 1950s, but recently numbers of cases have ↑ Rheumatic fever is still an endemic disease in developing countries *Peak incidence:* age 5–15y.

Cause: Rheumatic fever is due to an abnormal immunological response to β-haemolytic streptococcal infection (e.g. 2–4wk after sore throat). Its importance lies in the permanent damage caused to heart valves in some of those affected and subsequent risk of endocarditis.

Diagnosis: Can be made if revised Jones criteria are met (Table 3.8).

Management: If suspected refer for specialist care. Specialist management includes evaluation of heart lesions with echo, bed rest penicillin and symptom control (e.g. analgesia, sedatives for chorea) Anti-inflammatory agents such as corticosteroids and aspirin may be used to try to ↓ complications of carditis but their use is controversial.

Prognosis

- 60% develop chronic rheumatic heart disease (70% mitral valve; 40% aortic; 10% tricuspid; 2% pulmonary). Likelihood correlates with severity of initial disease.
- Recurrence may occur after further streptococcal infection or be precipitated by pregnancy or the COC pill.

2° prevention

- Penicillin 250mg bd po or sulfadiazine 1g od (500mg od for patients <30kg) for ≥5y. to prevent recurrence. Duration of prophylaxis is dependent on whether there was carditis in the initial attack (no carditis – continued for 5y.; if cardiac involvement – continued until age 25y. or longer).
- Once regular prophylaxis has stopped, patients should continue to have prophylactic antibiotics for dental and other operative procedures for life (Tables 3.6 & 3.7 – 📖 p.101).

Acute myocarditis: Inflammation of the myocardium. May present in a similar way to MI or with palpitations.

Causes

- Viral infection e.g. Coxsackie virus
- Diptheria
- Rheumatic fever
- Drugs

Management: Admit for specialist cardiologist care. Treatment is supportive. Some recover spontaneously – others progress to intractable heart failure requiring transplantation.

Table 3.8 Revised Jones criteria for diagnosis of rheumatic fever

Requirements for diagnosis of rheumatic fever

Evidence of previous streptococcal infection
(scarlet fever, +ve throat swab and/or ↑ ASO titre >200u/ml)

and

2 major criteria

or

1 major + 2 minor criteria

Major criteria	Minor criteria
Carditis (45–70%) – arrhythmia, new murmur, pericardial rub, heart failure, conduction defects.	Prolonged P–R interval on ECG (but not if carditis is one of the major criteria)
Migratory polyarthritis ('flitting' – 75%) red, tender joints.	Arthralgia (but not if arthritis is one of the major criteria)
Sydenham's chorea (St. Vitus' dance – 10%)	Fever
Subcutaneous nodules (2–20%)	↑ESR or ↑CRP
Erythema marginatum (2–10%)	History of rheumatic heart disease or rheumatic fever

Pericarditis and atrial myxoma

Acute pericarditis: Inflammation of the pericardium.

Presentation: Sharp, constant sternal pain relieved by sitting forwards. May radiate to left shoulder ± arm or into the abdomen. Worse lying on the left side and on inspiration, swallowing and coughing. A pericardial rub may be present at the left sternal edge on auscultation.

Causes

- Infection e.g. Coxsackie virus, TB
- Malignancy
- Uraemia
- MI (Dressler's syndrome 📖 p.72)
- Trauma
- Radiotherapy
- Connective tissue disease
- Hypothyroidism

Investigations: ECG – widespread, concave (saddle-shaped) ST elevation, PR segment depression – Figure 3.18.

Management: Refer to cardiology; treat the cause (if possible); symptomatic treatment with NSAID for pain; steroids in resistant cases.

Complications

Pericardial effusion: Fluid in the pericardial sac.

- *Presentation:* left or right heart failure, cardiac tamponade (inability of the heart to dilate in diastole resulting in tachycardia, ↓ BP, ↑ JVP). CXR – large, globular heart. Echo is diagnostic.
- *Management:* admit for urgent cardiology assessment.

Constrictive pericarditis: The pericardium becomes fibrosed and non-expansile. Most common cause is TB.

- *Presentation:* right heart failure, hepatosplenomegaly, ascites, ↓ BP, ↑ JVP.
- *Management:* refer to cardiology for confirmation of diagnosis. Treatment involves surgical release of the pericardium.

Atrial myxoma: Commonest primary cardiac tumour. Usually arises as a polypoid structure in the left atrium – less commonly in the right atrium/ventricles.

Presentation

- Breathlessness, blackouts/syncope, weight loss ± mild fever.
- Blood flow disturbance in the heart can result in thrombus formation and embolization (e.g. resulting in stroke).
- Examination may reveal a mid-diastolic murmur due to mitral valve obstruction by the tumour.

Investigations: ↑ ESR. Echo is diagnostic.

Management: Surgery is curative – refer.

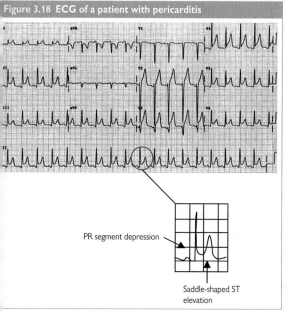

Figure 3.18 ECG of a patient with pericarditis

PR segment depression

Saddle-shaped ST elevation

Cardiomyopathy and heart transplant

Cardiomyopathy: Primary disease of the heart muscle.

Dilated (congestive) cardiomyopathy: Prevalence ≈35/100,00 population. ♂ > ♀. Dilation of left ± right ventricle and ↓ contractility. Presents with heart failure. ECG shows non-specific S–T abnormalities. CXR shows cardiac enlargement and pulmonary venous hypertension. Echo is diagnostic. *Causes:*

- Idiopathic
- Familial (20%)
- Cardiovascular – IHD, ↑BP, congenital heart disease, rheumatic heart disease
- Alcohol
- Infection e.g. Coxsackie virus, HIV
- Endocrine disease – myxoedema, thyrotoxicosis, acromegaly
- Cardiotoxic drugs
- Pregnancy
- Connective tissue disease (SLE, PAN, systemic sclerosis)
- Sarcoidosis
- Amyloidosis
- Haemachromatosis
- Malignancy
- Muscular dystrophy

Management and prognosis: Advise patients to stop drinking alcohol as alcohol may make the cardiomyopathy worse. Specialist management is needed in all cases and involves treatment of heart failure and arrhythmias. Most patients require long-term anticoagulation. Some need heart transplantation. *Mortality:* 40% in 2y. (sudden death, cardiogenic shock)

Hypertrophic cardiomyopathy: Familial inheritance (autosomal dominant) though 1:2 cases are sporadic. In its commonest form causes asymetrical septal hypertrophy ± aortic outflow obstruction (obstructive hypertrophic cardiomyopathy or HOCM).

Presentation: Most cases are diagnosed in childhood (<14y.) through screening of asymptomatic patients with a FH using echocardiography. *Symptoms/signs:*

- Palpitations – associated with arrhythmias – 5% have AF
- Breathlessness on exertion
- Chest pain – may be angina or atypical pain
- Murmur – due to outflow obstruction and/or mitral valve dysfunction
- Faints/collapses

Investigations:

- *ECG* – LVH and ischaemic changes e.g. T-wave inversion
- *CXR* – normal until disease is in its late stages
- *Echo* – diagnostic. Refer if suspicious symptoms or family history.

Management and prognosis: Ensure antibiotic prophylaxis for dental and other operative procedures (Tables 3.6 & 3.7 – 📖 p.101). Ongoing specialist care is essential to provide symptomatic treatment e.g. β-blockers for chest pain, amiodarone for arrhythmia (digoxin contraindicated). Surgical options include myotomy and myectomy.

Mortality: The major cause of mortality is sudden death which is unrelated to severity of symptoms. Though ultimately fatal in the majority interval between diagnosis and death is often decades.

Restrictive cardiomyopathy: Stiff ventricle which limits filling. Presents with heart failure. Echo is diagnostic. *Causes:* Amyloid, sarcoidosis, haemachromatosis. *Management:* Specialist management is required. Treatment is symptomatic.

Obliterative cardiomyopathy: Rare in Western countries – idiopathic fibrosis of inflow tract prevents filling and eventually leads to cavity obliteration.

Heart transplant: Considered in patients with estimated 1y. survival of <50%.

Indications/contraindications: Table 3.9

Assessment: Each eligible patient is assessed for psychosocial factors and physical factors (e.g. renal failure, obesity, age, peripheral vascular disease) which affect prognosis before a decision whether to place the patient on the transplant list is made.

Post-operatively: Patients require lifelong immunosuppression – usually with ciclosporine A. Follow-up is undertaken in specialist clinics.

Prognosis
- 1:4 patients die on the transplant list; 60% receive transplant in <2y.
- Perioperative mortality: <10%
- 1y. survival 92%; 5y. survival 75%; 10y. survival 60%
- Patients have accelerated graft atherosclerosis
- Complications of immunosuppression include ↑ risks of infection and cancer.

Table 3.9 Indications and contraindications for heart transplant   107

Indications	Contraindications
All patients must have end-stage heart disease. *Causes:*	Systemic disease likely to affect life expectancy (e.g. malignancy)
• IHD (50%)	Active infection (HIV, hepatitis B or C)
• Cardiomyopathy (40%)	Significant pulmonary vascular disease
• Valvular and congenital heart defects (5%)	Continued excess alcohol consumption
	Significant cerebral/systemic vascular disease
	Upper age limit is generally taken at ~60y.

Advice for patients: Patient information and support

Cardiomyopathy Association ☎01923 249 977
⌨ www.cardiomyopathy.org
Transplant Support Network ☎0800 027 4490/1
⌨ www.transplantsupportnetwork.org.uk
Heart Transplant Families Together ⌨ www.htft.org.uk

Congenital heart disease

Common, affecting ~6:1000 live births – Table 3.10.

Detection

Antenatal screening: Congenital heart disease may be detected *in utero* by USS. If detected during the routine 10–13wk. or 18wk. anomaly scan, amniocentesis is routinely offered to screen for Down's syndrome (~1:20 have heart disease – especially PDA, ASD and/or VSD) and other chromosomal abnormalities.

🚺 The exact nature of heart defects detected on antenatal USS is often not clear until birth – this can present parents with difficult decisions if there is any question of termination.

Examination: Neonatal examination detects ~44% of cardiac malformations detected <1y. of age. The rest are detected during routine developmental checks, if a murmur is detected incidentally when examining the child for another reason, or when the child becomes symptomatic.

Common presentations

Murmur on routine examination

- **Ventriculoseptal defect (VSD):** Harsh pansystolic murmur with splitting of the 2nd heart sound. Isolated VSD is the commonest congenital lesion in children (about 2:1000 births). Also occurs as a result of other complex lesions (e.g. Fallot's tetralogy).
- **Atrioseptal defect (ASD):** Systolic murmur in the pulmonary area with fixed splitting of the 2nd heart sound. May also present with heart failure or arrhythmia in a young adult.
- **Patent ductus arteriosus (PDA):** Loud, continuous 'machinery' murmur
- **Aortic stenosis:** Ejection systolic murmur at the apex & left sternal edge with a soft and delayed 2nd heart sound. Slow rising pulse, ↓BP. Rarely dizziness, faintness or loss of consciousness on exertion.
- **Pulmonary stenosis:** Ejection systolic murmur with ejection click.
- **Coarctation of the aorta:** Ejection systolic murmur over the left side and back; absent/delayed femoral pulses and upper limb hypertension.

🚺 **Innocent murmurs:** Murmurs are a common finding in childhood particularly when examining a febrile child. The majority are not associated with heart disease – so-called 'innocent murmurs'. *Features:*

- Asymptomatic
- Soft, systolic murmur – may vary with position and does not radiate
- Normal 2nd heart sound
- No other associated signs of heart disease (normal pulses, no thrill)

⚠ Unless a child is febrile when a murmur is heard – and the murmur disappears once afebrile – refer all children with murmurs for echo or paediatric evaluation.

Table 3.10 **Congenital cardiac abnormalities**	
Condition	Features
ASD	📖 p.118
Coarctation of the aorta	📖 p.118
Tetralogy of Fallot	Large VSD and pulmonary stenosis. In the newborn period may present with a murmur. Progressive cyanosis then develops over the next weeks/years ± ↓ exercise tolerance ± squatting after exercise. Treatment is surgical.
Hypoplastic left heart	Left ventricle ± mitral valve, aortic valve and aortic arch are underdeveloped. Presents within the 1st few days of life with heart failure. Treatment is surgical.
Patent ductus arteriosus (PDA)	The ductus arteriosus fails to close after birth. ♀>♂. Associated with prematurity. Symptoms depend on the size of the shunt. Presents with murmur ± failure to thrive ± heart failure. Treatment is usually surgical closure.
Transposition of the great arteries	The aorta arises from the right ventricle and the pulmonary artery from the left. Progressive cyanosis develops within a few hours of birth. Treatment is surgical.
Valve disease	📖 p.112
VSD	📖 p.120

109

ℹ Once a murmur has been assessed as being innocent, explain what that means to the parents – otherwise there may be unnecessary ongoing anxiety.

Advice for patients: A parent's experience of antenatal diagnosis

'Every time we went to the hospital we were told, "Well this is what we think is wrong." Which I know must be very, very difficult because at the end of the day they're scanning your baby through your tummy and it's very hard…Unfortunately for our daughter she couldn't have corrective surgery…But they still said to us, "Well we think this is the problem, but you know we may be not quite right, and when she's born we may be able to correct her heart depending on how certain things are." So when we were given the option of termination that was always in the back of our minds. Well how could we consider terminating a baby when the baby could have corrective heart surgery and everything could be fine? So we found that really, really hard.'

Heart failure
- Breathlessness, particularly when crying for feeding
- Failure to thrive
- Sweating
- Fast respiratory and pulse rates
- Heart enlargement
- Liver enlargement
- Weight increased due to fluid retention

Causes of heart failure in the 1st week of life include
- Left outflow obstruction
- Severe aortic stenosis
- Coarctation of the aorta
- Hypoplastic left heart

Later causes
- Large VSD
- PDA
- Ostium primum VSD

Cyanosis
- *<48h. old:* Likely to be due to transposition of the great arteries or severe pulmonary stenosis.
- *Later presentation:* Mostly due to *Tetralogy of Fallot* (Table 3.10, 📖 p.109).

Management: In all cases, if new congenital heart disease is detected, refer for specialist paediatric and/or cardiology opinion. Specialist treatment of valve lesions depends on the gradient measured across the valve. Most other congenital cardiac lesions (except VSD and ASD) require surgery – staged for complex lesions.

Prevention of endocarditis: An episode of endocarditis may be the presenting feature of congenital heart disease. There is ↑ risk of developing endocarditis in patients with valve lesions, septal defects (which persist after repair), PDA and particularly in those with prosthetic valves. All these patients require antibiotic prophylaxis for dental and surgical procedures – 📖 p.101.

Further information
Journal of the Royal College of Physicians of London Hunter *Congenital heart disease in adolescence* (2000) **34** (2) pp. 150–152
NEJM Brickner *et al. Congenital heart disease in adults* (2000) **342** (4) pp. 256–263

Advice for patients: Parents' experiences of diagnosis of congenital heart disease

Problems feeding

'Alex was born due to a normal delivery…She fed well and put on weight for the first two or three weeks of life and then she started to have problems feeding. I was breast-feeding at the time and I knew that there was something wrong…Health visitors and midwives didn't really pick up on it and felt that I was just having trouble breast-feeding …I tried bottle-feeding her and she continued not to put on weight … My health visitor said that it was because there was hot weather and things like that and not to worry… Towards the fifth week I was worried because she still hadn't put any more weight on from two weeks old. In fact she'd lost and I was very worried about this. So I took her to see the GP at 5 weeks old and my GP looked at her briefly, made a phone call to the hospital, sent me immediately up to the hospital and said that she could have a heart problem.'

Cyanosis

'And it all came to a head when she was four and a half months…and the little one, the baby, started with a cold so she was all runny nosed and very snuffly and not right at all … I managed to get an appointment. I didn't see our usual GP. I saw a female doctor who I hadn't seen before…and she said, "How long has she been like this?" I said, "What do you mean? She's got a cold, you know. The cold sort of started a couple of days ago but she's getting really snuffly." "No, how long has she been cyanosed?", which is blueness, and I said, "Oh she's been like this ever since she was born."… She said, "Well she's definitely cyanosed," and she sounded her chest and I could see the alarm bells ringing for her… And she said, "I want her to go hospital now."…And then he [the hospital doctor] said, "I think that she's in heart failure."'

Breathlessness

'We were on holiday…we noticed that she was quite breathless…We returned and I took my daughter to the doctor's, to my local GP … She checked her over and gave her some antibiotics for her chest infection, and she didn't alarm me at all but she asked me to come back the following week…We returned the following week and the doctor mentioned that she could hear a heart murmur and she said, "Don't be alarmed, it's found in many children. Don't worry about it but just to, you know, to have it double-checked, she needs to be referred to the hospital."…The doctor sounded her and he said yes that there was definitely a murmur there…and they took the ultrasound…and they said that [our daughter] had a hole in her heart.'

Information and support

Children's Heart Federation ☎ 0808 808 5000
🖳 www.childrens-heart-fed.org.uk

Valve disease

The heart valves can be come narrowed (stenosis) or leak (regurgitation). In both circumstances, the blood flow through the heart is disrupted and a murmur results. Other effects depend on which valve is affected and the degree to which the valve lesion affects the function of the heart as a pump.

Heart murmurs: 📖 p.32

Mitral regurgitation (incompetence): Common. *Causes:*

Primary: Due to valve disease.
- Mitral valve prolapse ('floppy mitral valve') – commonest cause
- Rheumatic fever – often other valve lesions too
- Ruptured papillary muscle/chordae tendinae following MI – sudden onset – may cause rapid heart failure
- Cardiomyopathy
- Connective tissue disease e.g. rheumatoid arthritis
- Endocarditis
- Congenital

Secondary: Due to dilation of the left ventricle e.g. due to heart failure, ischaemic heart disease (especially inferior MI), dilated cardiomyopathy.

Presentation
Symptoms: Dyspnoea, fatigue.

Signs
- Displaced apex (→ left axilla)
- Pansystolic murmur at the apex radiating to axilla
- AF
- Left ventricular failure

Management
- Confirm with echo
- Refer to cardiology – treatment is medical (digoxin and anti-coagulation for AF, diuretics) ± surgical (valve repair/replacement).
- Give antibiotic prophylaxis – 📖 p.101

Mitral valve prolapse: Prevalence ~1:20.

Presentation
Symptoms: Usually none. Rarely atypical chest pain, palpitations, syncope, postural hypotension, emboli.

Signs: Late systolic murmur over apex.

Management
- Confirm with echo.
- Antibiotic prophylaxis is needed for dental or surgical procedures if regurgitation or thickened (myxomatous) mitral valve leaflets (📖 p.101).
- If syncope or palpitations refer to cardiology – a rare complication is ventricular arrhythmia.

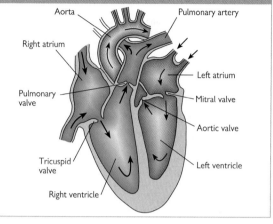

Figure 3.19 Cross section of the heart showing the heart valves and direction of blood flow

Aorta

Pulmonary artery

Right atrium

Left atrium

Pulmonary valve

Mitral valve

Aortic valve

Tricuspid valve

Left ventricle

Right ventricle

GP Notes:

Murmurs

- Benign functional murmurs are usually short and soft, and invariably systolic.
- Diastolic murmurs are always pathological.

Referral

⚠ All patients with newly detected valve disease, except those with mitral valve prolapse or aortic sclerosis, require cardiology referral.
- *Admit* if suspected endocarditis.
- *Refer urgently/admit* if symptomatic valve disease or if valve disease underlies the presenting condition e.g. heart failure caused by aortic stenosis, AF caused by mitral valve disease.

Mitral stenosis: Usually due to rheumatic fever.

Presentation
Symptoms
- Breathlessness
- Palpitations
- Fatigue
- May cause pulmonary hypertension which presents with right heart failure, haemoptysis and/or recurrent bronchitis.

Signs
- Peripheral cyanosis – 'malar flush' on cheeks
- Left parasternal heave
- Tapping apex beat
- AF
- Rumbling mid-diastolic murmur at the apex

Management
- Confirm with echo.
- Refer to cardiology.
- Treatment is medical (digoxin, diuretics, anticoagulation) ± surgical (valvotomy, balloon valvoplasty, valve replacement). Give antibiotic prophylaxis – 📖 p.101.

Aortic sclerosis: Senile thickening and stiffening of the aortic valve not associated with outflow obstruction. Clinically an ejection systolic murmur is present but no other symptoms or signs. CXR may show a calcified valve. No treatment is required.

Aortic stenosis: *Causes:*
- Degenerative calcification (commonest cause)
- Congenital e.g. bicuspid aortic valve (Figure 3.20 – common ~1:1000)
- Rheumatic fever
- Hypertrophic cardiomyopathy

Presentation
Symptoms: Angina, breathlessness, syncope or 'funny turns', dizziness, sudden death

Signs
- Small volume pulse with low pulse pressure (difference between systolic and diastolic BP).
- Ejection systolic murmur loudest in the aortic area which radiates to carotids and apex.

Management
- Echo is diagnostic and gives an estimate of gradient and thus severity.
- Refer to cardiology (urgently if symptomatic).
- Surgery (valve replacement or transcutaneous valvoplasty) is considered for those with symptoms or if systolic gradient across the valve is >50mmHg – even if the patient is elderly.
- Avoid treatment with ACE inhibitors.
- Give antibiotic prophylaxis – 📖 p.101.

Murmurs in pregnancy: Murmurs in pregnancy are very common and due to hyperdynamic circulation. Murmurs are usually soft and systolic. Loud murmurs are more likely to be pathological and diastolic murmurs are always abnormal.

Management: Consider any heart murmur detected during pregnancy significant and refer for further evaluation (e.g. with echo) – 90% will be physiological.

Pre-existing valve disease and pregnancy: Specialist obstetric care is required for all patients with a pre-existing cardiac condition. Where possible refer pre-conception to a cardiologist for discussion of risks. Women with valve disease require antibiotic prophylaxis for delivery – 📖 p.101.

Figure 3.20 Bicuspid and tricuspid aortic valves

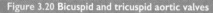
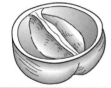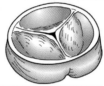

115

Further information
NEJM Carabello & Crawford *Medical progress: valvular heart disease* (1997) **337** pp. 32–41

Aortic regurgitation: Figure 3.21. *Causes:*

- Congenital e.g. VSD, bicuspid aortic valve
- Rheumatic fever
- Aortic dissection
- Endocarditis
- Cardiomyopathy
- Syphilis
- Marfan's or Ehlers–Danlos syndrome

Presentation
Symptoms: Dyspnoea, palpitations (extrasystoles)

Signs:
- Prominent pulse ('water-hammer') with wide pulse pressure
- Visible neck pulsation (Corrigan's sign)
- Head nodding in time with pulse (De Musset's sign)
- Visible capillary pulsations (e.g. in nail bed – Quincke's sign)
- Displaced apex beat
- High-pitched early diastolic murmur (easily missed)

Management
- Confirm with echo.
- Refer to cardiology for consideration of surgery.
- Give antibiotic prophylaxis – 📖 p.101.

Right heart valve disease

Tricuspid stenosis: Mitral valve disease always co-exists.
- *Cause:* rheumatic fever.
- *Murmur:* early diastolic (left sternal edge in inspiration).
- *Treatment:* diuretics ± surgery (valvotomy or replacement).

Tricuspid regurgitation: Figure 3.22
- *Causes:* right ventricular enlargement, endocarditis (IV drug abusers), carcinoid, rheumatic fever, congenital.
- *Presentation:* oedema, breathlessness, pulsatile hepatomegaly (± jaundice), ascites, and pansystolic murmur loudest at left sternal edge.
- *Treatment:* diuretics, vasodilators ± surgery (valve replacement or annuloplasty).

Pulmonary stenosis
- *Causes:* congenital (Fallot's tetralogy), rheumatic, carcinoid.
- *Murmur:* ejection systolic murmur (loudest to left of upper sternum, radiating to left shoulder).
- *Investigations: ECG:* Right ventricular hypertrophy; *CXR:* dilated pulmonary artery.
- *Treatment (if required):* pulmonary valvotomy.

Pulmonary regurgitation: Caused by pulmonary hypertension (📖 p.86)
Murmur: decrescendo early diastolic murmur at left sternal edge.

Management
- Echo is diagnostic in all cases.
- Always refer for specialist management.
- Give antibiotic prophylaxis – 📖 p.101.

Figure 3.21 Aortic regurgitation seen on colour flow doppler imaging

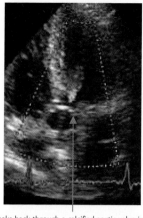

Blood leaks back through a calcified aortic valve in diastole

Figure 3.22 Tricuspid regurgitation

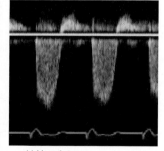

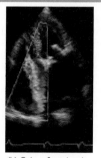

(a) M-mode image

(b) Colour flow doppler

Blood flow back through the tricuspid valve during systole

Other structural heart abnormalities

Coarctation of the aorta: Figure 3.23. Localized narrowing of the descending aorta usually distal to the origin of the left subclavian artery.

Presentation
- Heart failure
- ↑BP
- Murmur heard incidentally (ejection systolic murmur over the left side of the chest radiating to the back).
- Lack of femoral pulses or radio-femoral delay.
- Rarely presents with complications e.g. subarachnoid haemorrhage, endocarditis.

Investigations
- *CXR:* Prominent left ventricle.
- *ECG:* Left ventricular hypertrophy.

Management: Refer to cardiology – surgery to remove the narrowed portion of the aorta is usually indicated.

Atrial septal defect (ASD): A hole connects the 2 atria. Common – occurs in 2:1000 live births.
- Holes high in the septum (***ostium secundum***) are most common (Figure 3.24).
- Holes lower in the septum (***ostium primum***) are associated with atrio-ventricular valve abnormalities.

Blood flows from left → right through the shunt and the right heart takes the burden.

Presentation
Ostium secundum defects
- Symptoms are rare in infancy and uncommon in childhood. If detected in these groups presents as a murmur (systolic – loudest in the 2nd left interspace) found incidentally, or with breathlessness/tiredness on exertion, or recurrent chest infections.
- Presentation is usually in the 3rd or 4th decade with heart failure, pulmonary hypertension and/or atrial arrhythmias.

Ostium primum defects: Heart failure commonly develops in infancy childhood ± severe pulmonary hypertension. In addition to the ASD murmur, there may be a pansystolic murmur signifying mitral or tricuspid valve regurgitation.

Investigation
- *CXR:* Cardiomegaly with a prominent right atrium ± pulmonary artery ± pulmonary plethora.
- *ECG:* Right axis deviation (ostium secundum defect) or left axis deviation (ostium primum defect), right ventricular hypertrophy ± RBBB.
- *Echo:* Diagnostic.

Management: Refer to cardiology. Cardiac surgery to close the defect i usually indicated. Mortality from percutaneous repair is low. Give all patient with ostium primum defects prophylactic antibiotics – 📖 p.101.

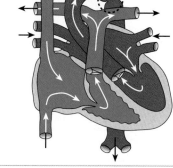

Figure 3.23 Coarctation of the aorta

Narrowing of the aorta:
BP is ↑ in the vessels
which leave the aorta
above this point

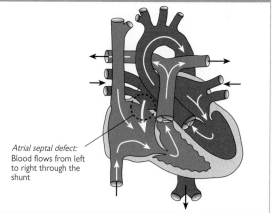

Figure 3.24 Ostium secundum atrial septal defect

Atrial septal defect:
Blood flows from left
to right through the
shunt

GP Notes: ASD, VSD or Marfan syndrome and pregnancy

Specialist obstetric care is required for all patients. Where possible, refer pre-conception to a cardiologist for discussion of risks. Antibiotic prophylaxis is necessary for women with ostium primum ASDs, VSDs or valve lesions – 📖 p.101.

Figures 3.23 and 3.24 are reproduced from the *Report of the Manitoba pediatric cardiac surgery inquest* with permission.

Ventricular septal defect (VSD): A hole connects the 2 ventricles (Figure 3.25). Blood flows initially from left → right through the hole. May be congenital or acquired.

Congenital VSD

Small VSD ('maladie de Roger'): Normally asymptomatic.
- *Examination:* Thrill palpable at lower left sternal border; harsh pansystolic murmur – small holes give loud murmurs.
- *Investigations:* CXR and ECG are normal. Diagnosis is confirmed on echo.
- *Management:* Refer to cardiology – usually surgery is not indicated.

Moderate VSD: Symptoms usually appear in infancy – breathlessness on feeding/crying, failure to thrive, recurrent chest infections. As the child gets older symptoms improve (relative size of the defect ↓).
- *Examination:* Cardiomegaly, thrill palpable at left sternal edge, pansystolic murmur.
- *Investigations:* CXR: cardiomegaly ± prominent pulmonary arteries ± pulmonary plethora. Diagnosis is confirmed on echo.
- *Management:* Refer to cardiology – surgery is indicated if the child is not improving or there is evidence of pulmonary hypertension.

Large VSD: Presents with heart failure at ~3mo. of age though there may be symptoms of breathlessness on feeding/crying prior to this.
- *Examination:* Baby is obviously unwell – underweight, breathless, pulmonary oedema ± cyanosis, large heart, thrill over left sternal edge ± parasternal heave, murmur – often not pansystolic due to high right ventricular pressures.
- *Management:* Admit to paediatrics – medical treatment ± surgery is always needed.

Acquired VSD: Usually due to septal rupture post-MI. Suspect if new pansystolic murmur ± heart failure develop after MI. Investigate as for congenital VSD. Refer to cardiology for advice on further management – urgency of referral depends on the clinical state of the patient.

⚠ All patients with VSD require prophylactic antibiotics (📖 p.101).

Marfan syndrome: Autosomal dominant connective tissue disease causing abnormalities of fibrillin (a glycoprotein in elastic fibres). Features include:
- Arachnodactyly (long spidery fingers)
- High-arched palate
- Arm span > height
- Lens dislocation ± unstable iris
- Aortic dilatation (β-blockers appear to slow this)
- Aortic incompetence can develop e.g. in pregnancy
- Aortic dissection may cause sudden death – echo screening may be helpful for affected individuals.

If suspected refer to cardiology ± genetics.

Other congenital heart disease: 📖 p.108

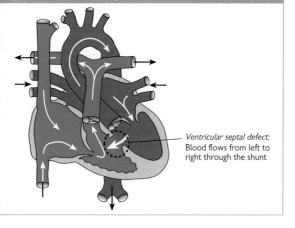

Figure 3.25 Ventricular septal defect

Ventricular septal defect:
Blood flows from left to
right through the shunt

121

Figure 3.25 is reproduced from the Report of the *Manitoba pediatric cardiac surgery inquest* with permission.

Acute stroke

Common and devastating condition – most common cause of adult disability in UK. ½ all strokes occur in people >70y.

Definitions
- **Stroke:** Syndrome typified by rapidly developing signs of focal or global disturbance of cerebral functions, lasting >24h. or leading to death, with no apparent causes other than of vascular origin. (WHO 1978)
- **Transient ischaemic attack (TIA)** or 'mini-stroke': neurological symptoms resolve in <24h.

Causes
- **Cerebral infarction** (≈70%): Atherothrombotic occlusion or embolism. *Sources of embolism*: left atrium (AF) or left ventricle (MI or heart failure). Ischaemia causes direct injury from lack of blood supply.
- **Intracerebral or subarachnoid haemorrhage** (≈19%): Haemorrhage causes direct neuronal injury and pressure exerted by the blood results in adjacent ischaemia.
- **Rare causes:** Sudden ↓BP, vasculitis, venous-sinus thrombosis, carotid artery dissection.

Risk factors
- Age
- ↑BP
- DM
- AF
- Previous stroke or TIA
- Previous MI
- Artificial heart valves
- Hyperviscosity syndromes
- Smoking
- Alcohol
- Obesity
- Low physical activity

Presentation
- **History:** Sudden onset of CNS symptoms, or stepwise progression of symptoms over hours or days.
- **Examination:** Conscious level may be ↓ or normal; neurological signs (including dysphagia and incontinence); BP; heart rate and rhythm; heart murmurs; carotid bruits; systemic signs of infection or neoplasm.

Differential diagnosis
- Decompensation after recovery from a previous stroke (e.g. due to infection, metabolic disorder)
- Space occupying lesion – 1° or 2° cerebral neoplasm, cerebral abscess
- Trauma – subdural haematoma, traumatic brain injury
- Other neurological conditions e.g. epileptic seizure, migraine, MS

Acute management
- Admit all patients who have suffered an acute stroke to hospital.
- Do not give aspirin prior to admission.
- Treatment of stroke in a stroke unit → ↓ mortality and morbidity[C].
- All patients should have a CT/MRI scan <48h. after admission to demonstrate the site of the lesion, distinguish between ischaemic and haemorrhagic stroke and identify conditions mimicking stroke.
- Recent evidence regarding benefits of thrombolysis means acute admission bypassing the GP altogether will be the norm in future[C].

GMS contract

Stroke 1	The practice can produce a register of patients with stroke or TIA	2 points	
Stroke 11	% of new patients with a stroke who have been referred for further investigation	up to 2 points	40–80%

GP Notes: After a stroke

Stroke is a family illness

- 40% of informal carers (usually spouse or close relative) suffer psychological distress 1 year after the stroke.
- Involve carers and families.
- Provide information and support.

Stroke is a devastating illness for the patient. Address psychosocial issues as well as physical disability.

Monitor and reassess frequently

- Continue follow-up even when specialist services have finished. Stroke is a long-term problem.
- Monitor secondary prevention measures (📖 p.126).
- Refer for more specialist rehabilitation if there is any deterioration in function.
- Remember aids and appliances can help and patients and carers might be entitled to benefits (📖 p.225).

Concordance with medication – after stroke most patients will be prescribed ≥1 drugs to ↓ their risk of further stroke, but some have memory loss or problems opening containers. All patients should receive verbal and written information about their medicines and receive help with packaging e.g. non-childproof tops.

Advice for patients: Information and support for patients and carers

Stroke Association ☎ 0845 30 33 100 🖥 www.stroke.org.uk
Northern Ireland Chest, Heart and Stroke Association
☎ 0845 76 97 299 🖥 www.nichsa.com
Chest, Heart and Stroke Association Scotland 🖥 www.chss.org.uk
Different Strokes ☎ 0845 130 7172 🖥 www.differentstrokes.co.uk
Speakability ☎ 0808 808 9572 🖥 www.speakability.org.uk

Transient ischaemic attack (TIA): Presents with a history o
sudden-onset focal neurological deficit – usually maximal at onset
Recovery takes place within 24h. of initial symptoms. The most com
mon focal deficits are:

- motor symptoms (e.g. hemiparesis or weakness)
- speech or language problems (e.g. dysphagia, dyslexia or dysarthria)
- sensory symptoms (e.g. visual or somatic sensory symptoms).

Non-focal symptoms are non-specific and may be due to other causes
They include:

- Light-headedness
- Feeling faint
- Blackouts
- Confusion.

⚠ Patients with a history of TIA have a 20% risk of stroke in the
following month with highest risk in the first 72h. – see Table 3.11

Investigations

- ECG
- CXR
- Blood – FBC, ESR, U&E, Cr, lipids, glucose
- Consider clotting screen ± thrombophilia screening if FH thrombosis

Management of TIA

- Once all symptoms have stopped, start aspirin 50–300mg od.
- Start treatment for risk factors e.g. advise to stop smoking, start
  antihypertensives if ↑ BP.
- Refer for assessment and further investigation to a specialist service
  e.g. neurovascular clinic. The National Stroke Guidelines state that al
  patients with a history of TIA should be seen in a specialist clinic <7d
  after the event. Specialist investigations include: CT or MRI scan to
  confirm diagnosis, carotid dopplers if carotid artery territory
  symtoms echocardiogram if recent MI, CCF/LVF or murmur.
- Admit if >1 TIA within 1 wk.

Amaurosis fugax: A form of TIA due to emboli passing throug
the retina. Causes brief loss of vision (few minutes) 'like a curtain
Management is as for TIA (See above).

Further information

Royal College of Physicians National clinical guidelines for stroke
(2nd edition, 2004) 🖳 www.rcplondon.ac.uk
BMJ Bath & Lees ABC of arterial and venous disease: acute stroke (2000)
320 p. 920–923.

Cochrane Reviews

- Organised inpatient (stroke unit) care for stroke Stroke Unit Trialists'
  Collaboration (2002)
- Thrombolysis for acute ischaemic stroke Wardlaw et al. (2003)

NICE Guidance on management of stroke due to be published in 2008

Table 3.11 The ABCD scoring system predicts future risk of stroke after TIA

ABCD	Feature	Score
Age	<60y.	0
	≥60y.	1
BP	Systolic >140 and/or diastolic ≥90	1
Clinical features	Unilateral weakness	2
	Speech disturbance without weakness	1
	Other	0
Duration	≥60min.	2
	10–59min.	1
	<10min.	0

- ABCD scores of 5 or 6 carry a 24% chance of stroke in <7d.
- Patients with a score <5 have a 0.4% chance of stroke in <7d.

Table 3.11 is reproduced from the *Lancet*, Rothwell, P.M., *et al.* A simple score (ABCD) to identify individuals at high early risk of stroke after a transient ischaemic attack (2005) **366:** 9479, pp.29–36., with permission from Elsevier.

Secondary stroke prevention

Patients with a past history of stroke or TIA/amaurosis fugax have a 30–43% risk of recurrent stroke within 5y.

Prevention focuses on ischaemic/embolic events which account for the majority of strokes. *Strategies include:*

Lifestyle advice
- Stopping smoking[£]
- Regular exercise
- Diet (low fat, high fibre, include plant sterols) and achieving a satisfactory weight
- Reducing salt intake
- Avoiding alcohol excess – predisposes to both ischaemic and haemorrhagic stroke through effects on BP.

Antiplatelet drugs (usually aspirin)[£]
- All patients not taking warfarin, who have suffered a non-haemorrhagic stroke (confirmed on CT/MRI) or a TIA, should be started on aspirin as soon as possible after the event.
- Aspirin ↓ long-term risks of cardiovascular events by ¼ .
- *Dose of aspirin*: 50–300mg od for maintenance therapy.
- Dipyridamole 200mg bd can be used in addition to aspirin (effects are additive).
- Clopidogrel 75mg od is an expensive alternative to aspirin. Use if unable to tolerate aspirin.

⚠ For patients with suspected stroke DON'T start aspirin prior to admission.

Warfarin
1° *prevention*
- Patients who have identified potential causes of cardiac thromboemboli should be anticoagulated with warfarin. This includes patients with:
  - Rheumatic mitral valve disease
  - A prosthetic heart valve
  - Dilated cardiomyopathy *and*
  - AF associated with valvular heart disease or prosthesis.
- Anticoagulate patients with non-valvular AF *only* if annual risk of stroke is >3% (Table 3.12). If < 3%, start aspirin instead.

2° *prevention*[£]
- *All* patients who have suffered a stroke or TIA and have persistent or paroxysmal AF or a major source of cardiac embolism should be anticoagulated with warfarin.
- Start >14d. after stroke and only if haemorrhagic stroke has been excluded.
- Target INR 2–3 if no other indication.

Table 3.12 Non-valvular AF and stroke

Risk group	Annual risk of stroke		
	Untreated	Aspirin	Warfarin
Very high Previous ischaemic stroke/TIA or thrombo-embolic event	12%	10%	5%
High Age ≥75y. with ↑BP, DM or vascular disease Clinical evidence of valve disease or heart failure Left ventricular dysfunction on Echo	5–8%	4–6%	2–3%
Moderate Age ≥65y. no high risk factors Age <75y. ↑BP, DM and/or vascular disease	3–5%	2–4%	1–2%
Low Age <65y. with no moderate, high or very high risk factors	1.2%	1%	≈0.5%

High or very high risk – anticoagulate with warfarin unless contraindications. Target INR 2–3, if contraindications, treat with aspirin 75–300mg od.

Moderate risk – aspirin (75–300mg od) or anticoagulation with warfarin (target INR 2–3) are both options. Take into account patient preference and weight risks against benefits of anticoagulation for each patient. Stroke risks are cumulative so if ≥ 1 moderate risk factor (e.g. DM and ↑ BP) then benefits of anticoagulation increase.

Low risk – treat with aspirin 75–300mg od

GMS contract

Stroke 1	The practice can produce a register of patients with stroke or TIA	2 points	
Stroke 12	% of patients with a stroke shown to be non-haemorrhagic, or history of TIA, with a record that an anti-platelet agent (aspirin, clopidogrel, dipyridamole or a combination), or an anticoagulant is being taken (unless contraindication or side-effects recorded)	up to 4 points	40–90%

Smoking targets: 📖 p.249

Hypertension management[£]

- Systolic and diastolic BP independently predict stroke. Risk escalates with increasing BP. 5–6mmHg ↓BP reduces risk by >30%.
- National Stroke Guidelines recommend treatment with a combination of a thiazide diuretic and ACE inhibitor. Aim to keep systolic BP <140mmHg and diastolic BP <85mmHg (<130/80 if diabetic).
- After stroke (but not after TIA) defer treating hypertension until >2wk. after the event as ↑BP may be physiological response – lowering BP decreases perfusion of the brain and may be harmful.

Cholesterol

1° prevention

- Analysis of data from the coronary prevention trials shows a 22% ↓ cholesterol using a statin produces a 30% ↓ in stroke in individuals with no past history of stroke/TIA.
- Treat with a statin (e.g. simvastatin 40mg od) if diabetic or 10y. cardiovascular disease (CVD) risk ≥20%[G].
- Risk can be estimated with tables (Figures 4.1 and 4.2, 📖 p.154–155) and computer programmes e.g. *Coronary heart disease event* and *Stroke risk calculator* (download free from the British Hypertension Society website 🖥 www.bhsoc.org).

2° prevention[£]

- There is evidence to suggest all patients with a history of CVD should be treated with a statin regardless of baseline cholesterol[G].
- National Stroke Guidelines suggest treatment with a statin e.g. simvastatin 40mg od if diabetic or total cholesterol is >3.5 mmol/l unless contraindicated.

Treatment target: Aim to ↓ total cholesterol by 25% or to <4mmol/l whichever is the lower value *or* to ↓ LDL cholesterol by 30% or <2.0 mmol/l – whichever is the lower value.

Carotid stenosis and carotid endarterectomy: Carotid endarterectomy ↓ mortality if carotid stenosis is symptomatic. Benefits decrease as the degree of stenosis gets smaller – there is no evidence of benefit <30% stenosis.

- *Patients with asymptomatic stenosis:* There is a 2% annual risk of stroke so the place of surgery is controversial; in general, risks outweigh benefits, so start aspirin and ↓ other modifiable risk factors.
- *Patients with a history of stroke/TIA:* Referral for carotid endarterectomy or carotid artery stenting should be considered for any patients who:
  - have a history of stroke/TIA
  - have >70% carotid artery stenosis *and*
  - do NOT have severe disability.

Vaccination[£]: Patients disabled due to stroke are at risk from pneumococcal infection and influenza. Make sure they are offered vaccination.

> ### Advice for patients: Information and support for patients and carers
>
> **Stroke Association** ☎ 0845 30 33 100 🖥 www.stroke.org.uk
> **Northern Ireland Chest, Heart and Stroke Association**
> ☎ 0845 76 97 299 🖥 www.nichsa.com
> **Chest, Heart and Stroke Association Scotland** 🖥 www.chss.org.uk

GMS contract

Stroke 1	The practice can produce a register of patients with stroke or TIA	2 points	
Stroke 5	% of patients with TIA/stroke who have a record of blood pressure in the notes in the preceding 15mo.	up to 2 points	25–90%
Stroke 6	% of patients with a history of TIA/stroke in whom the last reading (measured in last 15mo.) is ≤150/90	up to 5 points	25–70%
Stroke 7	% of patients with TIA/stroke who have a record of total cholesterol in the last 15mo.	up to 2 points	25–90%
Stroke 8	% of patients with TIA/stroke whose last measured total cholesterol (measured in last 15mo.) was ≤5mmol/l	up to 5 points	25–60%
Stroke 10	% of patients with TIA/stroke who have had influenza immunization in the preceding 1st September – 31st March	up to 2 points	25–85%

Hypertension targets: 📖 p.253
Influenza and pneumococcal vaccination: may be offered by GMS practices as a directed enhanced service – 📖 p.260.

129

Further information
Royal College of Physicians National clinical guidelines for stroke (2nd edition, 2004) 🖥 www.rcplondon.ac.uk
BMJ Bath et al. ABC of arterial and venous disease: secondary prevention of TIA and stroke (2000) **320** pp. 991–995
NICE Atrial fibrillation: the management of atrial fibrillation (2006) 🖥 www.nice.org.uk
JBS2 Joint British Societies' guidelines on prevention of cardiovascular disease in clinical practice (2005). Heart **91** (Suppl. 5): v1–52

Aneurysms

An arterial aneurysm forms when there is a >50% ↑ in the normal diameter of the vessel. Aneurysms may affect any medium/large artery aorta/iliac arteries > popliteal > femoral > carotid. Family history of aneurysm is a risk factor.

Causes
- Atheroma (commonest)
- Injury
- Infection e.g. endocarditis, syphilis – mycotic aneurysms

Abdominal aortic aneurysm (AAA): Aneurysmal dilatation of the aorta in the abdomen. Prevalence 5% and increasing. The typical patient with an AAA is a ♂ smoker >65y. Risk ↑ x4–10 if there is an affected 1st degree relative. Screening and management – 📖 p.132.

Thoracoabdominal aneurysm: Involves thoracic and abdominal aorta, including the origins of the visceral and renal arteries. Surgery more complex than that for AAA and carries higher mortality. Management – see opposite.

Popliteal aneurysms: 80% peripheral aneurysms. Most are >2cm diameter; 50% are bilateral. Associated with AAA (40%).

Presentation: Acute below knee ischaemia $2°$ aneurysm thrombosis or embolization. Popliteal pulses are pronounced. Diagnosis is confirmed on USS.

Management
- Acute ischaemia – 📖 p.135.
- Elective surgery (popliteal bypass) – when aneurysm >2.5cm diameter.

Femoral artery aneurysms: *Presentation:* local pressure symptoms, thrombosis or distal embolisation. *Surgical treatment:* bypass surgery.

Cerebral artery aneurysms: Berry aneurysms may run in families and are associated with polycystic kidneys, coarctation of the aorta and Ehlers-Danlos syndrome.

Presentation: Subarachnoid haemorrhage. Typically presents as a sudden devastating headache – 'thunderclap headache' – often occipital. Rarely (6%) preceded by a 'sentinel headache' representing a small leak ahead of a larger bleed. Vomiting and collapse with loss of consciousness ± fitting ± focal neurology follow.

Examination: May be nothing to find initially. Neck stiffness takes 6h. to develop. In later stages:
- Papilloedema
- Retinal and other intraocular haemorrhages
- Focal neurology
- ↓ level of consciousness

Action: If suspected admit immediately as a medical emergency. Only 1:4 admitted with suspected SAH turn out to have one. In most no cause for the headache is found.

Dissecting thoracic aneurysm

- Consider in any patient with ↓BP and chest pain – especially if the pain radiates through to the back.
- Typically presents with sudden tearing chest pain radiating to the back.
- As the dissection progresses, branches of the aorta are sequentially occluded causing:
  - Hemiplegia – carotid artery
  - Unequal pulses and BP in the two arms – subclavian artery
  - Paraplegia – spinal arteries
  - Acute renal failure – renal arteries.
- Proximal extension may cause aortic incompetence and MI due to occlusion of the cardiac arteries.

Management

- Obtain venous access with 2x large-bore IV cannulae.
- Admit as 'blue light' emergency, keeping the patient flat in the ambulance.
- Warn relatives of poor prognosis.

Advice for patients: Information and support for patients and carers

Circulation Foundation ▯ www.circulationfoundation.org.uk
Vascular Society of GB & Ireland ▯ www.vascularsociety.org.uk

Abdominal aortic aneurysm

Abdominal aortic aneurysm (AAA) is common. Prevalence is ~5% an increasing. The typical patient with an AAA is a ♂ smoker >65y. Risk x4–10 if there is an affected 1st degree relative.

Screening

- Acute rupture of AAA in the community has ~90% mortality rate.
- Elective surgical repair has ~5–7% mortality.
- Single abdominal USS in men age 65y. would exclude 90% of the population from future AAA rupture.
- A large RCT of population screening in the UK showed 44% ↓ in death due to AAA in the screened group over 4y.
- Trials evaluating cost-effectiveness of screening have suggested that screening smoking ♂ at 65y. may be more cost-effective.
- Decisions on population screening are awaited. Meanwhile consider screening men with IHD and ↑BP – especially if smokers.

Problems with screening: Identifies small aneurysms not requiring repa but surveillance. This may cause morbidity in low risk, healthy individual

Presentation of AAA: Often discovered as an incidental finding o abdominal examination, X-ray (calcification of aneurysm wall in 50% cases) or USS (¾ asymptomatic at diagnosis). Otherwise presents with
- *Local symptoms* – vague abdominal or back pain
- *Distant symptoms* – embolization/acute ischaemia of a limb. Multiple small infarcts (e.g. of toes) with good peripheral pulses suggest an aneurysm proximally
- *Acute rupture* – see opposite.

Investigation: USS confirms diagnosis, diameter, site and extent.

Management of

- *Acute rupture* – see opposite.
- *Referral for elective surgery*
  - Refer if risk of rupture > risk elective repair.
  - The greater the diameter, the more the risk (5.5cm diameter ≈10% 1y. rupture rate; 10cm diameter >75% 1y. rupture rate).
  - AAAs >5.5cm are routinely repaired unless other factors ↑ risk o surgery. There is no survival benefit treating smaller aneurysms.
  - Refer urgently if symptomatic – may indicate rapid expansion or inflammation – both risk factors for rupture.
- *USS surveillance:* Patients with AAAs <5.5cm diameter. Annual screening. Routine repair takes place when and if the aneurysm expands to >5.5cm. 3:5 eventually warrant surgery.

Inflammatory aneurysms: Characterized by inflammatory infiltrat in the aneurysm wall. May be adherent to surrounding structure *Presentation:* fever, malaise and abdominal pain. Associated with ↑ mo tality at operation.

Ruptured abdominal aortic aneurysm

- In the community setting, death rate from ruptured AAA ≈90% – 80% die before reaching hospital and 50% that get to hospital die during surgery.
- Consider a ruptured AAA in any patient with ↓BP and atypical abdominal symptoms (especially if there is a pulsatile abdominal mass).

Management

- Obtain venous access with 2x large-bore IV cannulae.
- Admit as 'blue light' emergency, keeping the patient flat in the ambulance.
- Warn relatives of poor prognosis.

⚠ In a patient with a known AAA, abdominal pain represents a ruptured AAA unless proven otherwise.

GP Notes: Factors predisposing to rupture of AAA

- Diameter (risk ↑ with diameter)
- COPD
- Smoking
- ↑ diastolic BP
- Family history
- Fast rate of expansion
- Inflammation within the aneurysm wall
- Thrombus-free surface area of aneurysm sac

Advice for patients: Information and support for patients and carers

Circulation Foundation 🖥 www.circulationfoundation.org.uk
Vascular Society of GB & Ireland 🖥 www.vascularsociety.org.uk

133

Further information

British Heart Foundation Factfiles *Abdominal aortic aneurysms* (03/2003) 🖥 www.bhf.org.uk

Peripheral ischaemia

Chronic peripheral ischaemia: Peripheral vascular disease (normally atherosclerotic) commonly affects arteries supplying the legs. *Incidence:* 10% patients age 60–70y.; 20% >70y.

Natural history: Most remain stable. A few (2% over 10y.) progress from intermittent claudication to critical limb ischaemia. Management of cardiovascular risk factors is essential.

Intermittent claudication: Restriction of blood flow causes pain on walking.

Risk factors

- ♂ > ♀
- Smoking
- Obesity
- ↑BP
- Hyperlipidaemia
- DM
- Physical inactivity
- Hypercoagulable states
- Postmenopausal

Presentation: Presents with muscular, cramp-like pain in the calf, thigh or buttock on walking that is rapidly relieved on resting. The leg is cool and white with atrophic skin changes and absent pulses:

- *Disease in the superficial femoral artery* – absent popliteal and foot pulses. Causes calf claudication.
- *Disease of the aorta or iliac artery* – weak or absent femoral pulse ± femoral bruit. Causes calf, thigh or buttock claudication.

Differential diagnosis: Nerve root compression e.g. sciatica; spinal stenosis – usually bilateral pain which may occur after prolonged standing as well as exercise – not rapidly relieved by rest.

134

Investigation

- *Blood:* FBC, U&E, Cr (peripheral vascular disease is associated with renal artery stenosis), glucose, lipids.
- *Ankle-brachial systolic pressure index (ABPI):*
  - Good history + ABPI < 0.95 confirms diagnosis
  - If good history but normal ABPI (=1), consider exercise testing*.
- *Duplex USS:* Used to determine site of disease*.

Management

- **↓ risk factors:** Patients with claudication have a 3x ↑ risk of death from MI/stroke. Advise to stop smoking and lose weight. Ensure optimum treatment of ↑BP, lipids and DM.
- **Foot care:** Regular chiropody.
- **Drugs:**
  - Aspirin (75–300mg od) ↓ risk of cardiovascular events. Alternatives are dipyridamole (200mg bd) or clopidogrel (75mg od).
  - Naftidrofuryl – may ↑ walking distance – unclear whether influences outcome. Reassess after 3–6mo. Discontinue if no improvement.
  - Cilostazol – ↑ walking distance in those with ongoing symptoms despite risk factor management.
- **Exercise:** Training for ≥6mo. by regularly walking as far as possible before being stopped by pain, ↑ pain-free and maximum walking distances. Effect is greater than the effect of angioplasty.

* May only be available via 2° care referral.

Acute limb ischaemia

Causes

- Acute thrombotic occlusion of pre-existing stenotic segment (60%)
- Embolus (30%)
- Trauma e.g. compartment syndrome or traumatic vessel damage

Presentation

- Pain
- Pallor
- Paraesthesia
- Pulselessness
- Paralysis
- Perishing cold

Management: Admit acutely under the care of a vascular surgeon. Treatment can be surgical (e.g. embolectomy) or medical (e.g. thrombolysis).

GP Notes: Referral to vascular surgery

- Critical limb ischaemia – E/U
- Severe symptoms – S
- Job affected – S/R
- Uncertainty about diagnosis – R
- No better after exercise training – R

E = Emergency admission; U = Urgent; S = Soon; R = Routine

Advice for patients: Information and support for patients and carers

Circulation Foundation ⬚ www.circulationfoundation.org.uk

The diabetic foot: 📖 p.164

Critical limb ischaemia

Presentation: Deteriorating claudication and nocturnal rest pain (usually just after fallen asleep – hanging the foot out of bed improves the pain). Ulceration or gangrene results from minor trauma.

Examination: Look for:
- Atrophic skin changes – pallor, cool to the touch, hairless, shiny
- On lowering the leg turns a dusky blue–red colour; on elevation – pallor and venous guttering.
- Ulceration – check under the heel and between the toes
- Swelling suggests the patient is sleeping in a chair to avoid rest pain or, rarely, pain from deep infection
- Absent foot pulses – if present consider alternative diagnosis
- ABPI <0.5 – 🛈 arterial calcification can result in falsely high readings.

Management: Analgesia (often requires opiate); refer for urgent vascular surgical assessment.

Specialist management
- *Angiography:* To assess extent and position of disease.
- *Percutaneous transluminal angioplasty ± stenting:* Most suitable for short occlusions/stenoses of the iliac and superficial femoral vessels. 1y. patency rate 80–90%.
- *Surgery:* Most suitable for longer occlusions/multiple stenoses – aortobifemoral bypass grafts have 5y. patency rates >90%; femoropopliteal bypass grafting gives 5y. patency rates of <70%. Aspirin ↓ risk of re-occlusion. Amputation is a last option.

Further information

British Heart Foundation Factfiles *Peripheral vascular disease* (09/2001) 🖥 www.bhf.org.uk
Journal of Vascular Surgery Dormandy & Rutherford *Management of peripheral arterial disease* (2000) **31** p. S1–S296
NEJM Hiatt WR *Medical treatment of peripheral arterial disease and claudication* (2001) **344** pp. 1608–1621

| DM 9 | % of patients with diabetes with a record of presence or absence of peripheral pulses in the previous 15mo. | up to 3 points | 40–90% |

Erectile dysfunction

Persistent inability to obtain or maintain sufficient rigidity of the penis to allow satisfactory sexual performance. Frequently due to vascular disease.

Incidence/prevalence: 50% men aged 40–70y. experience some degree of erectile dysfunction – always ask – incidence is ↑:

- x2 in hypertensives – consider changing medication if onset of erectile dysfunction is within 2–4wk. of initiation of drug therapy e.g. thiazides
- x3 in patients with DM
- x4 in men with established coronary artery disease – more likely to have multi-vessel than single-vessel coronary artery disease
- x2 in smokers.

Risk factors: Smoking, ↑BP, hyperlipidaemia, DM, excessive alcohol

History: Ensure the presenting problem is erectile dysfunction and not other sexual difficulties; identify risk factors (see above).

Examination and investigation

- Testosterone insufficiency – ↓ libido – measure morning testosterone – refer to endocrinology if hormone abnormalities.
- Peripheral vascular disease – peripheral pulses.
- Psychological distress – mental state.
- Check BP, fasting lipid profile and glucose.

GP management: Counsel the couple about the problem, its possible causes and management – Figure 3.26.

- Advice on lifestyle – ↓ smoking and alcohol. Weight loss and ↑ exercise for obese, underactive patients improves both sexual function and cardiovascular health.
- Discuss pros and cons of available drug treatment. Phosphodiesterase type 5 inhibitors (PDE5s) are the mainstays of treatment – titrate dose to effect (most diabetics need the maximum dose); warn the patient he may need 8 attempts before a satisfactory erection occurs. Side-effects include headache, flushing and acid reflux.
- Review progress – adjust dosage, consider other treatment options (intraurethral/intracavernosal alprostadil, vacuum devices) and/or referral to urologist.

Table 3.13 PDE5 inhibitors and action times

Drug	Onset of action in min. (*Peak action*)	Duration of action in h.	Doses
Sildenafil	20–30 (*60*)	4–6	25–50–100mg
Tadalafil	60–120 (*120*)	36–48	10–20mg
Vardenafil	20–30 (*60*)	4–6	5–10–20mg

⚠ PDE5 inhibitors are contraindicated for patients taking nicorandil or nitrates.

Further information

British Heart Foundation Factfile *Drugs for erectile dysfunction* (06/2005) available from 🖳 www.bhf.org.uk

Table 3.13 is reproduced from British Heart Foundation Factfile *Drugs for erectile dysfunction* (06/2005). Available from 🖳 www.bhf.org.uk

Figure 3.26 Algorithm for management of erectile dysfunction

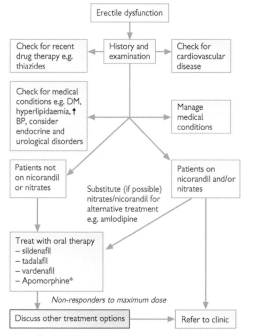

*not as effective as PDE 5 inhibitors but not contraindicated with nitrates

GP Notes:

⚠ All men >25y. with erectile dysfunction should be screened for cardiac risk factors and signs or symptoms of vascular disease.

ⓘ NHS prescriptions for impotence are available **only** for men:
- treated for prostate cancer, with kidney failure, spinal cord injury, DM, MS, spina bifida, Parkinson's disease, polio, severe pelvic injury or who have had radical pelvic surgery or a prostatectomy
- already receiving drug treatment for impotence on 14.09.98
- through specialist services for men suffering severe distress due to impotence.

Endorse FP10/GP10 with SLS.

Figure 3.26 is reproduced from British Heart Foundation Factfile *Drugs for erectile dysfunction* (06/2005). Available from 🖳 www.bhf.org.uk

Varicose veins

Anatomy: Figure 3.27. The veins of the legs are divided into 2 systems:
- The deep veins run deep to the muscle fascia
- The superficial veins run in the subcutaneous fat layer.

In a number of places in the leg, the superficial and deep veins are linked by perforating veins (or 'perforators').

What are varicose veins? Tortuous, twisted or lengthened veins.

Primary varicose veins: Most varicose veins are primary. The vein wall is inherently weak causing dilatation and separation of valve cusps so they become incompetent. Blood flows backwards from the deep to superficial venous system, causing back pressure and further dilatation.

Risk factors: Age, parity, occupations requiring a lot of standing, obesity (women only).

Secondary varicose veins: Due to ↑ pressure in the venous system due to DVT, pelvic tumour, pregnancy or A–V fistula.

Prevalence: 17–31%. ♂ > ♀ (≈5:4).

Assessment: *Consider:*
- *Why is the patient consulting now?* Patients are often worried about appearance of varicose veins or prognosis if left untreated but have no other symptoms attributable to the veins (1:3 consultations).
- *Symptoms:* Heaviness, tension, aching (worse on standing and in the evening; improved by elevating the leg and support stockings), itching.
- *Complications:* See below.
- *PMH:* Previous surgery or injection for varicose veins, pregnancy, past history of DVT or thrombophlebitis, COC pill or HRT.
- *FH:* Varicose veins or DVT.

Examination
- *Abdominal examination:* To exclude 2° causes.
- *Veins:* With the patient standing, inspect distribution of the veins and any 2° skin changes. Patterns of distribution (Figure 3.27):
  - *Long saphenous distribution:* thigh and medial aspect of the calf.
  - *Short saphenous distribution:* below the knee on the posterior and lateral aspects of the calf.

Complications
- Haemorrhage
- Varicose eczema – Figure 3.31, 📖 p.143
- Skin pigmentation – Figure 3.31, 📖 p.143
- Oedema
- Thrombophlebitis
- Venous ulceration – 40% don't have visible varicose veins – Figure 3.32, 📖 p.143
- Atrophie blanche – white, lacy scars
- Lipodermatosclerosis – fibrosis of the dermis and subcutis around the ankle → firm induration

Figure 3.27 Veins of the leg

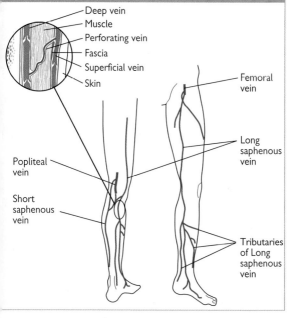

- Deep vein
- Muscle
- Perforating vein
- Fascia
- Superficial vein
- Skin

Femoral vein

Long saphenous vein

Popliteal vein

Short saphenous vein

Tributaries of Long saphenous vein

GP Notes: Tredelenberg test – used to establish site of valvular incompetence in patients with varicose veins

1. Ask the patient to lie down.
2. Elevate the leg.
3. Empty the veins by massaging distally to proximally.
4. Block the superficial veins in the upper thigh using a tourniquet.
5. Ask the patient to stand up.
6. If the tourniquet stops the veins rapidly refilling, the incompetent valve must be higher i.e. at the sapheno-femoral junction. If they refill, the communication must be lower.
7. Apply the tourniquet at intervals down the leg until it controls refilling:
   - above the knee – to assess the mid-thigh perforator
   - below the knee – to assess competence between the short saphenous and popliteal veins.
8. If refilling can't be controlled, communication is probably via distal perforating veins.

gure 3.27 is reproduced with modifications from 🖳 www.familydoctor.co.uk

Table 3.14 Grading of varicose veins

Grade	Appearance	Symtoms/Complication
Grade 1	Spider veins Star bursts Thread veins Matted veins Intradermal venules <1mm Reticular veins – dilated tortuous subcutaneous veins not belonging to the main branches of the long or short saphenous vein	Unsightly but otherwise asymptomatic.
Grade 2	Varicose veins	*Symptoms* Aching Tingling Cramps Itching Heaviness Swelling Restless legs Cosmetic *Complications:* None
Grade 3	Varicose veins with skin changes at the ankle	*Symptoms:* As for grade 2 veins *Complications:* Oedema Venous eczema Superficial phlebitis
Grade 4	Varicose veins with more widespread skin changes attributed to venous disease	*Symptoms:* As for grade 2 veins *Complications:* Oedema Venous eczema Lipodermatosclerosis Superficial phlebitis Venous ulceration
Grades 5 & 6	Late-stage venous disease	Severe skin changes and/or active ulceration

Figure 3.28 Grade 1 varicose veins

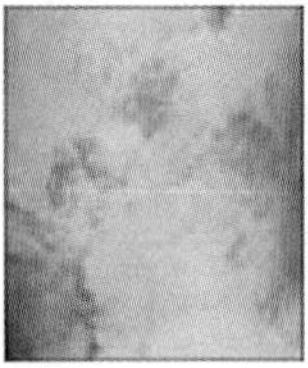

Permission to reproduce Table 3.14 and Figure 3.28 sought from Frimley Park Hospital NHS Foundation Trust.

Figure 3.29 Grade 2 varicose veins: unsightly veins but no secondary skin changes or complications

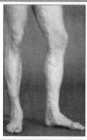

Figure 3.30 Grade 3 varicose veins: mild skin discolouration at the ankle

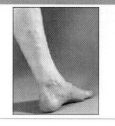

Figure 3.31 Grade 4 varicose veins: varicose eczema, widespread skin discolouration and atrophie blanche

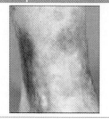

143

Figure 3.32 Venous ulcer

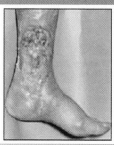

Management: Reassurance is often all that is needed.
- *If symptoms are troublesome:* Advise:
  - Support stockings
  - Avoid standing for prolonged periods
  - If standing don't stand still
  - Walk regularly
  - ↓ weight if obese.
- *If any complications or severe symptoms:* Refer for surgical assessment. In general, patients with purely cosmetic problems are not treated under the NHS.

Bleeding varicose veins: Bleeding can be stemmed by raising the foot above the level of the heart and applying compression. If the patient is fit for surgery, refer for surgical assessment. Once recovered from the bleed, advise compression hosiery.

COC pill and HRT: Women with varicose veins taking the COC pill or HRT are not at ↑ risk of DVT but are at ↑ risk of thrombophlebitis.

Saphena varix: Dilatation of the saphenous vein at its confluence with the femoral vein which transmits a cough impulse. May have bluish tinge and disappears on lying down. A cause of a lump in the groin (differential diagnosis – Table 3.15). Action only needed if symptomatic.

Thrombophlebitis: Presents as severe pain, erythema, pigmentation over, and hardening of the vein. Thrombophlebitis in varicose veins results from stasis. Consider underlying malignancy or thrombophilia if thrombophlebitis occurs in normal veins or there is recurrent thrombophlebitis in varicose veins.

Management: There is no indication for antibiotics.
- Crepe bandaging to compress vein and minimize propogation of thrombus
- Analgesia – preferably NSAID
- Ice packs and elevation
- Low dose aspirin – 75–150mg od

⚠ If phlebitis extends up the long saphenous vein towards the sapheno femoral junction, refer for urgent duplex scanning – saphenofemoral ligation may be indicated if thrombus extends into the femoral vein.

Follow-up: If the patient is fit for surgery, refer for surgical assessment as thrombophlebitis tends to recur if the underlying venous abnormality is not corrected.

ⓘ History of thrombophlebitis is a contraindication to the COC pill and a reason to stop for current users. Evidence regarding HRT is less clear.

Thrombophlebitis migrans: Recurrent tender nodules affecting veins throughout the body. Associated with carcinoma of the pancreas

Table 3.15 Differential diagnosis of groin lumps

Position relative to the skin	Groin lump	Position relative to the inguinal ligament	
		Above	Below
In the skin	Lipoma, fibroma, haemangioma and other skin lumps	✓	✓
Deep to the skin	Femoral or inguinal lymph nodes	✓	✓
	Saphena varix of the femoral vein	✗	✓
	Femoral artery aneurysm	✗	✓
	Femoral hernia	✗	✓
	Inguinal hernia	✓	✗

🛈 The inguinal ligament runs from the pubic tubercle medially to the anterior superior iliac spine laterally.

Advice for patients: Information for patients and carers

Circular Foundation 🖥 www.circulationfoundation.org.uk

Deep vein thrombosis (DVT)

Any deep vein can clot. Common sites are the limbs, mesentery, cerebral sinus and retina. Deep vein thrombosis in the leg (commonest site) may be proximal – involving veins above the knee – or isolated to the calf veins. *Incidence:* 1:1000 people/y. in developed countries.

Risk factors:

- Age 40y.
- Smoking
- Obesity
- Immobility
- Recent long distance travel
- Pregnancy
- Puerperium
- COC pill/HRT use
- Surgery

- Recent trauma
- Malignancy
- Heart failure
- Nephrotic syndrome
- Inflammatory bowel disease
- Past medical history of thromboembolism
- Inherited clotting disorder
- Other chronic illness

Presentation: Unilateral leg pain, swelling and/or tenderness ± mild fever, pitting oedema, warmth and distended collateral superficial veins

Differential diagnosis

- Cellulitis
- Haematoma
- Ruptured Baker's cyst
- Superficial thrombophlebitis
- Chronic venous insufficiency
- Venous obstruction

- Post-thrombotic syndrome
- Acute arterial ischaemia
- Lymphoedema
- Fracture
- Hypoproteinaemia

Immediate action: Clinical diagnosis is unreliable.

- Only 50% of DVTs are symptomatic.
- <50% with clinically suspected DVT have diagnosis confirmed on diagnostic imaging.

Refer all suspected DVTs for further assessment. Many hospitals have rapid access to facilities for diagnosis, bypassing conventional admission

Specialist assessment: Clinical probability scores are used to decide whether patients fall into high or low probability groups for DVT.

- *If low probability:* A blood D-dimer test is done (detects a degradation product of fresh venous thrombus). If the D-dimer test is –ve, DVT is excluded. If +ve, the patient is assessed as if medium/high probability.
- *If medium/high probability:* USS assessment is undertaken.
  - If USS is negative and low probability or -ve D-dimer, DVT is excluded.
  - If USS is positive, diagnosis of DVT is confirmed.
  - If USS is negative but medium/high probability or +ve D-dimer, USS is repeated after 1 wk. or the patient is assessed with venography, CT or MRI.

GP Notes:

Long-haul flights and DVT: DVT is very rare in this situation. Aspirin is not indicated. Advise patients to:
- Drink plenty of non-alcoholic fluids
- Keep their legs moving whilst sitting, or walk up and down the aisle.

Graduated compression hosiery is available for purchase OTC and does ↓ risk of DVT. Recommended for all long-haul flights and particularly for patients who are taking the COC pill, have a chronic illness e.g. inflammatory bowel disease, have recently undergone surgery, or are relatively immobile.

Those with a history of DVT during flight need heparin cover – refer for specialist advice.

Thrombophilia^G: ↑ tendency to clot. The commonest genetic factor is Leiden factor V (about 5% of population) which increases risk of venous thromboembolism x8. Antithrombin deficiency (1:5,000) confers a 50% risk of venous thromboembolism aged <50y.

Screening for clotting tendency: Test blood for Leiden factor V if:
- Venous thromboembolism <45y.
- Arterial thrombosis <40y.
- Recurrent thromboembolism/thrombophlebitis
- Unexplained prolonged partial thromboplastin time
- Clear family history of venous thrombosis
- Family history of thrombophilic abnormality
- Patients with systemic lupus erythematosis, idiopathic thrombocytopoenic purpura or recurrent foetal loss
- Skin necrosis (especially if on warfarin)
- Unexplained neonatal thrombosis.

Management: Refer to haematology. Patients may need short-term prophylaxis with anticoagulants at times of risk (e.g. surgery, pregnancy) or rarely long-term anticoagulation.

Further information

British Committee for Standards in Haematology Diagnosis and management of heritable thrombophilia (2001)
🖳 www.bcshguidelines.com

Management of patients with confirmed DVT

- Initial anticoagulation is with low-molecular-weight heparin (LMWH) followed by oral anticoagulation (warfarin) – usually as an out-patient
- LMWH should be continued for at least 4d. and until INR is in the therapeutic range for ≥2d. Target INR is 2.5 (range 2–3).
- Oral anticoagulants ↓ risk of further thromboembolism and should be continued for 3–6mo. after a single DVT (🕮 p.158).
- Graduated elastic compression stockings – should be worn for >2y. as they ↓ risk of post-thrombotic leg syndrome by 12–50%.

Isolated calf DVT: There is some debate whether anticoagulation is necessary. Untreated 40–50% extend to proximal DVT and anticoagulation ↓ risk extension. Some specialists prefer to treat with compression stockings and follow with serial USS.

Management of DVT during pregnancy[G]:
Pregnancy ↑ risk of thromboembolism x 10. Thromboembolism complicates ≈1:100 pregnancies (20–50% antenatal). Suspect DVT and/or PE in any woman who is pregnant or in the puerperium who has pain or swelling in the leg, mild unexplained fever, chest pain and/or breathlessness.

Risk factors
- Caesarean section
- Prolonged bed rest
- Previous thromboembolism
- Antiphospholipid syndrome (below)

Management: Refer for expert advice.
- Warfarin is teratogenic when used in the 1st trimester of pregnancy and can increase miscarriage, maternal and fetal haemorrhage, and stillbirth rates. Avoid during pregnancy. LMWH is a safe alternative.
- Warfarin is safe post-partum and during breast–feeding.

Prevention: Prophylaxis is required if a patient has a thrombophilia (🕮 p.147) or past history of pregnancy or COC pill-associated thromboembolism. LMWH is used antenatally and for up to 6wk post-partum – refer for expert advice.

Antiphospholipid syndrome:
Antiphospholipid antibodies (lupus anticoagulant and/or anti-cardiolipin antibodies) and a history of ≥1 of:
- arterial thrombosis
- venous thrombosis
- recurrent pregnancy loss (typically 2nd trimester).

Can be 1° (occurs alone) or 2° to another connective tissue disease usually systemic lupus erythematosis.

Associated with:
- ↑ risk of thrombosis
- ↑ risk of pre-eclampsia
- ↑ pregnancy loss – causes ~20% of recurrent miscarriages; <20% pregnancies result in live birth.

Management: Specialist referral is essential. Treatment is with aspirin or LMWH throughout pregnancy.

Further information

Royal College of Obstetricians and Gynaecologists

📖 www.rcog.org.uk

Thromboprophylaxis during pregnancy, labour and after vaginal delivery (2004)

Thromboembolic disease in pregnancy and the puerperium (2001)

Complications of DVT

Post-thrombotic syndrome: Occurs after DVT. Results in chronic venous hypertension causing limb pain, swelling, hyperpigmentation, dermatitis, ulcers, venous gangrene and lipodermatosclerosis.

Recurrent venous thromboembolism: Patients with history of thromboembolism have ↑ risk of recurrence in high-risk situations (e.g. trauma, surgery, immobility, pregnancy) and should receive prophylaxis with heparin/oral anticoagulants in such situations.

Pulmonary embolus (PE): Venous thrombi – usually from a DVT – pass into the pulmonary circulation and block blood flow to the lungs. Without treatment 20% with proximal DVT develop PE. Fatal in ~1:1 cases causing ~20,000 deaths/y. in UK hospitals.

Risk factors
* Immobility – long flight or bus journey, post-op, plaster cast
* Smoking
* COC pill
* Pregnancy or puerperium
* Malignancy
* Past history or family history of DVT or PE

Presentation
* *Symptoms:* Acute dyspnoea, pleuritic chest pain, haemoptysis, syncope.
* *Signs:*
  * Hypotension
  * Tachycardia
  * Cyanosis
  * Tachypnoea
  * Pleural rub
  * ↑JVP
* Look for a source of emboli – though often DVT is not clinically obvious.

⚠ Have a high level of suspicion. Patients may have minimal symptoms/signs apart from some pleuritis pain and dyspnoea. PE in the community can be linked with surgical procedures done 2–3 wk. previously.

Differential diagnosis
* Pneumonia and pleurisy
* MI/unstable angina
* Other causes of acute breathlessness – acute LVF, asthma, exacerbation of COPD, pneumothorax, shock (e.g. due to anaphylaxis), arrhythmia, hyperventilation
* Other causes of acute chest pain – aortic dissection, rib fracture, musculoskeletal chest pain, pericarditis, oesophageal spasm, shingles

Immediate action: If suspected, give oxygen as soon as possible and admit as an acute medical emergency.

Specialist management: Involves investigation to prove diagnosis (ventilation–perfusion [VQ] scan, MRI and/or pulmonary angiography). Thrombolytic therapy is controversial but usually given for major (life-threatening) PEs. In all cases of proven PE, anticoagulation is started. Warfarin should be continued for 6mo., aiming to keep the INR ≈ 2.5 (range 2–3).

Chapter 4

Management of risk factors for cardiovascular disease

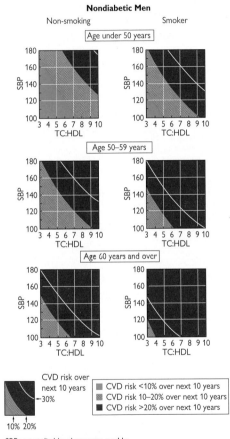

Figure 4.1 CVD risk chart–non-diabetic men

Nondiabetic Men

Non-smoking · Smoker

Age under 50 years

Age 50–59 years

Age 60 years and over

CVD risk over next 10 years

■ CVD risk <10% over next 10 years
■ CVD risk 10–20% over next 10 years
■ CVD risk >20% over next 10 years

SBP = systolic blood pressure mmHg
TC:HDL = serum total cholesterol to HDL cholesterol ratio

⚠ These charts are not appropriate for use with patients with pre-existing CHD, familial hypercholesterolaemia, chronic renal dysfunction, or DM.

Figure 4.1 is reproduced with permission © The University of Manchester.

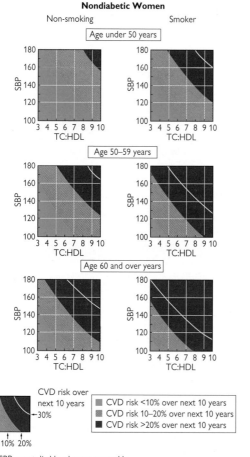

Figure 4.2 CVD risk chart–non-diabetic women

Nondiabetic Women

Non-smoking   Smoker

Age under 50 years

Age 50–59 years

Age 60 and over years

CVD risk over next 10 years
~30%
10% 20%

CVD risk <10% over next 10 years
CVD risk 10–20% over next 10 years
CVD risk >20% over next 10 years

SBP = systolic blood pressure mmHg
TC:HDL = serum total cholesterol to HDL cholesterol ratio

Patients in the following groups have ↑ risk:
• Family history of premature CHD or stroke (multiply risk by 1.5x)
• Originate from the Indian subcontinent (multiply risk by 1.5x)
• ↑ triglycerides, premature menopause, or impaired glucose tolerance.

Aspirin for prevention of vascular disease

Antiplatelet therapy is effective in ↓ cardiovascular morbidity and mortality. Aspirin (75–300mg od for maintenance treatment; 150–300mg for acute stroke/MI) is the agent most widely used. For patients with contraindications to aspirin, clopidogrel (75mg od) is an expensive alternative.

Cautions
- Risk of major GI bleed at aspirin doses of 75–300mg od is 1:500 patient-years. ↓ gastric intolerance by using 75mg od, using dispersible or enteric-coated preparations, PPIs or H$_2$ receptor antagonists.
- Avoid concomitant use of warfarin except on specialist advice as it significantly ↑ risk of bleeding.

Indications
Coronary heart disease[£]
1° prevention – advise for 1° prevention of MI in adults:
- With DM if ≥50y., DM for >10y. and/or receiving treatment for ↑ BP
- If >50y. and 10y. cardiovascular disease (CVD) risk ≥20%.

75mg od results in a 20% ↓ in non-fatal MI at a cost of a small ↑ in risk of bleeding. Benfit ↑ with ↑ absolute risk of CHD.

2° prevention – advise for 2° prevention if:
- Suspected acute MI or unstable angina (start dose 150–300mg)
- Previous MI, angina, coronary artery surgery or angioplasty

↑ BP: Patients age ≥50y. with satisfactory BP control (<150/90mmHg) + target organ damage, DM or 10y. CVD risk ≥20%.

Target organ damage: Heart failure, established CHD, stroke/TIA, peripheral arterial disease, abnormal renal function (↑ Cr or proteinuria/microalbuminuria), hypertensive or diabetic retinopathy, left ventricular hypertrophy on ECG or Echo.

Stroke[£]: Following ischaemic stroke/TIA or carotid endarterectomy. Warfarin is preferable for patients with AF or other causes of cardioembolic stroke.

Peripheral arterial disease: Patients with claudication, peripheral angioplasty or arterial grafts.

AF: Risk factors for stroke: previous ischaemic stroke/TIA, ≥65y., ↑ BP, DM, cardiac failure, value disease, Echo showing LV dysfunction or mitral valve calcification.
- If AF, <65y and no additional risk factors – given aspirin 75–300 mg od.
- If AF, ≥65y or ≥1 risk factor – consider treatment with warfarin in preference to aspirin – 📖 p.127.

GMS contract				
CHD 9	% of patients with coronary heart disease with a record in the last 15 mo. that aspirin, an alternative anti-platelet therapy, or an anticoagulant is being taken (unless a contra-indication or side-effects are recorded)	7 points	40–90%	
Stroke 12	% of patients with a stroke shown to be non-haemorrhagic stroke, or history of TIA, with a record that an antiplatelet agent (aspirin, clopidogrel, dipgridamole or a combination) or anticoagulant is being taken (unless a contraindication or side-effects are recorded)	up to 4 points	40–90%	
AF 3	% of patients with AF who are currently treated with anti-coagulant or anti-platelet drug therapy	up to 15 points	40–90%	

Anticoagulation

Heparin in the community: Only use on specialist advice. Usually s/cut low-molecular-weight (LMW) heparin used as it does not need daily monitoring.

Warfarin: Acts by antagonizing the effects of vitamin K and thus ↓ clotting tendency. It takes 48–72h. for anticoagulant effect to develop fully so not used initially when acute effect is required. Indications and target INRs – Table 4.1.

Initiation of warfarin

- *Acute anticoagulation (e.g. PE):* Admit to hospital for heparinization then warfarinization with heparin cover.
- *For DVT:* Anticoagulation is often started in the community with heparin and then warfarin under specialist direction.
- *If no urgency (e.g. chronic AF):* Warfarin can be started in the community. Check baseline blood sample for FBC, clotting screen, urea and liver function tests. Complete a DoH oral anticoagulant booklet for the patient to carry. Take patients (or carers) through the educational do's and don'ts in the booklet. Advise that the daily dose of warfarin should be taken at a fixed time.

Dose regime for starting warfarin in the community: Table 4.2 (📖 p.160).

Monitoring: Table 4.3 (📖 p.160). If there is a change in clinical state monitor more frequently until steady state is re-established. Have an explicit system for handling results promptly, making informed decisions on further treatment and testing, and communicating results to patients. Monitor the process with regular audit.

Self-monitoring

Consider if preferred by the patient and:

- Patient/carer is physically and cognitively able to perform the self-monitoring test.
- An adequate educational programme is in place to train patients/carers.
- Equipment is regularly checked.
- Ability to self-manage is regularly reviewed.

Recurrent arterial thrombosis/embolism on anticoagulants

Seek specialist advice. *Consider:*

- Compliance
- Modifiable risk factors – smoking, ↑BP, lipids
- Cardiac sources of emboli (echo)
- Thrombophilias (📖 p.147)
- Arteritis e.g. collagen disorders, syphilis
- Malignant disease

Further information

SIGN Antithrombotic therapy (1999) 🖥 www.sign.ac.uk
British Journal of Haematology Guidelines on oral anticoagulation (3rd edition – 1999) **101** p. 374–387 🖥 www.bcshguidelines.com

Table 4.1 Indications for oral anticoagulation and target INR

Indication	Target INR (target range)	Duration of treatment
Cardiac		
Mechanical prosthetic heart valves		
1st generation	3.5 (3.0–4.0)	Long term
2nd generation	3.0 (2.5–3.5)	
Rheumatic mitral valve disease	2.5 (2.0–3.0)	Long term
Valvular AF and AF due to congenital heart disease or thyrotoxicosis	2.5 (2.0–3.0)	Long term
Non-valvular AF and medium/high risk of stroke (📖 p.127)	2.5 (2.0–3.0)	Long term
Dilated cardiomyopathy	2.5 (2.0–3.0)	Long term
Mural thrombus post-MI	2.5 (2.0–3.0)	3 mo.
Cardioversion	2.5 (2.0–3.0)	3wk. before procedure and for 4wk. after procedure
Venous thromboembolism		
1st PE/proximal vein thrombosis and no persistent risk factors	2.5 (2.0–3.0)	6 mo.
1st calf vein thrombosis and no persistent risk factors	2.5 (2.0–3.0)	3 mo.
Prophylaxis of recurrent DVT/PE		
occurring on warfarin	3.5 (3.0–4.0)	Long term
occurring off warfarin	2.5 (2.0–3.0)	
Other disorders		
Inherited thrombophilia with no previous thrombosis	2.5 (2.0–3.0)	Anticoagulate for high-risk activities e.g. surgery
Inherited thrombophilia with previous episode of thrombosis	2.5 (2.0–3.0)	Long term
Antiphospholipid syndrome	2.5–3.5	Long term

⚠ Warfarin is a dangerous drug:
- It causes numerous admissions every year with bleeding.
- It interacts with a large number of drugs, including aspirin, some antibiotics, cimetidine, corticosteroids, and NSAIDs.
- It is teratogenic.

Table 4.2 is reproduced with permission from *British Journal of Clinical Pharmacology*, (1998); **46** 157–61.

Table 4.2 Dose regime for starting warfarin in the community

INR on day 5	Dose days 5–7	INR on day 8	Dose from day 8
≤1.7	5mg	≤1.7	6mg
		1.8–2.4	5mg
		2.5–3	4mg
		>3	3mg for 4d.
1.8–2.2	4mg	≤1.7	5mg
		1.8–2.4	4mg
		2.5–3	3.5mg
		3.1–3.5	3mg for 4d.
		>3.5	2.5mg for 4d.
2.3–2.7	3mg	≤1.7	4mg
		1.8–2.4	3.5mg
		2.5–3	3mg
		3.1–3.5	2.5mg for 4d.
		>3.5	2mg for 4d.
2.8–3.2	2mg	≤1.7	3mg
		1.8–2.4	2.5mg
		2.5–3	2mg
		3.1–3.5	1.5mg for 4d.
		>3.5	1mg for 4d.
3.3–3.7	1mg	≤1.7	2mg
		1.8–2.4	1.5mg
		2.5–3	1mg
		3.1–3.5	0.5mg for 4d.
		>3.5	omit for 4d.
>3.7	0mg	<2	1.5mg for 4d.
		2–2.9	1mg for 4d.
		3–3.5	0.5mg for 4d.

Instructions:
- Give warfarin 5mg od for 4d. then check INR.
- Adjust dose as in table.
- Recheck INR on day 8 and adjust dose as in table.
- Thereafter check INR weekly (unless 4d. interval stated) and adjust dose accordingly until dose is stable in the target range.

⚠ **High INR**

INR ≥8 (lower if other risk factors for bleeding) – admit to hospital even if not bleeding.

INR >3.7 and <8 – omit warfarin 1–2d. and recheck INR. Restart when INR <5 and re-titrate dose.

Table 4.3 Warfarin therapy: recall periods during maintenance therapy

INR	Recall interval and action
1 INR high ⚠ If INR>8 – admit	Recall 7–14d. Stop treatment for 1–3d. (max 1wk. in prosthetic valve patients) and restart at a lower dose.
1 INR low	↑ dose and recall in 7–14d.
1 therapeutic INR	Recall 4wk.
2 therapeutic INRs	Recall 6wk. (maximum interval if prosthetic heart valve).
3 therapeutic INRs	Recall 8wk.*
4 therapeutic INRs	Recall 10wk.*
5 therapeutic INRs	Recall 12wk.*

* Except prosthetic heart valves where maximum recall interval is 6wk.

CHD 9	% of patients with coronary heart disease with a record in the last 15mo. that aspirin, an alternative antiplatelet therapy, or an anticoagulant is being taken (unless a contraindication or side-effects are recorded)	7 points	40–90%
Stroke 12	% of patients with a stroke shown to be non-haemorrhagic or history of TIA, with a record that an antiplatelet agent (aspirin, clopidogrel, dipyridamole or a combination) drug, or anticoagulant is being taken (unless a contraindication or side-effects are recorded)	up to 4 points	40–90%
AF 3	% of patients with AF who are currently treated with anti-coagulant or anti-platelet drug therapy	up to 15 points	40–90%
Records 9	For repeat medicines, an indication for the drug can be identified in the records (for drugs added to the repeat prescription with effect from 01.04.2004)	4 points	Minimum standard 80%

Anticoagulation monitoring may be provided by practices as a national enhanced service – 📖 p.261.

Diabetes and cardiovascular disease

> ⚠ **Don't use arterial risk tables for adults with DM**

Diabetics are at ↑ risk of MI (2–5x), stroke (2–3x) and peripheral vascular disease. Protective effect of female gender is lost. Atherosclerotic disease accounts for most of the excess mortality due to DM. Check arterial risk factors annually:
- Albumin excretion rate[£]
- Blood glucose control[£]
- BP[£]
- Lipid profile (LDL, HDL cholesterol and triglycerides)[£]
- Central obesity
- Smoking[£] – give advice on cessation at every opportunity – 📖 p.188.

Metabolic syndrome: Consists of impaired glucose tolerance or DM insulin resistance + other disorders of ↑ cardiovascular risk including:
- Central obesity – waist circumference ≥88cm (♀) or ≥102cm (♂). For Asian population use waist circumference ≥80cm (♀) or ≥90cm (♂).
- Dyslipidaemia – fasting triglyceride >1.7mmol/l (non-fasting >2.0mmol/l) and/or HDL cholesterol <1.0mmol/l (♂) or <1.2mmol/l (♀)

ⓘ Patients have a very high risk of cardiovascular disease – treat all risk factors aggressively.

Impaired glucose tolerance: Risk factor for DM and cardiovascular disease. Follow up with annual fasting glucose – 4%/y. develop DM Treat cardiovascular risk factors aggressively.

Aspirin: Give 75mg od to type 1 and type 2 diabetics:[G]
- with atherosclerotic disease and/or
- if ≥50y. and/or
- if DM for >10y. and/or
- who are receivng treatment for ↑ BP

ⓘ Control systolic BP to ≤145mmHg before starting treatment.

Statin[£]

If aged ≥ 40y.: Prescribe statin to all type 1 and type 2 diabetics[G].

If aged 18–36y.: Prescribe statin if ≥1 of:
- retinopathy – pre-proliferative, proliferative, maculopathy
- nephropathy, including persistent microalbuminuria
- poor glycaemic control – HbA1c >9%
- ↑ BP requiring antihypertensive therapy
- ↑ total blood cholesterol ≥6.0 mmol/l
- features of metabolic syndrome (see above)
- family history of premature CVD in first degree relative (men <55y.: women <65y.).

Aim to
- ↓ total cholesterol by 25% or to <4mmol/l – whichever is lower *or*
- ↓ LDL cholesterol by 30% or to <2.0mmol/l – whichever is lower.

GMS contract			
DM 19	The practice can produce a register of patients aged ≥17y. with DM which specifies whether the patient has type 1 or type 2 DM	6 points	
DM 2	% of patients with DM whose notes record body mass index in the previous 15 mo.	up to 3 points	40–90%
DM 5	% of patients with DM who have a record of HbA_{1c} or equivalent in the previous 15mo.	up to 3 points	40–90%
DM 20	% of patients with DM with HbA_{1c} ≤7.5 (or equivalent test/reference range depending on local laboratory) in the previous 15mo.	up to 17 points	40–50%
DM 7	% of patients with DM with HbA_{1c} ≤10 (or equivalent test/reference range depending on local laboratory) in the previous 15mo.	up to 11 points	40–90%
DM 11	% of patients with DM who have a record of BP in the previous 15mo.	up to 3 points	40–90%
DM 12	% of patients with DM in whom the last BP is ≤145/85	up to 18 points	40–60%
DM 13	% of patients with DM who have a record of micro-albuminuria testing in the previous 15mo. (exception reporting if proteinuria)	up to 3 points	40–90%
DM 16	% of patients with DM who have a record of total cholesterol in the previous 15mo.	up to 3 points	40–90%
DM 17	% of patients with diabetes whose last measured total cholesterol within the previous 15mo was ≤5mmol/l	up to 6 points	40–70%

Coronary heart disease: p.245
Hypertension: p.253
Smoking: p.249

Advice for patients: Information and support
Diabetes UK ☎ 0845 120 2960 🖳 www.diabetes.org.uk

Further information

BS2 Joint British Societies' guidelines on prevention of cardiovascular disease in clinical practice (2005). *Heart* 91 (Suppl. 5): v1-52
NICE 🖳 www.nice.org.uk
• Type 1 diabetes: diagnosis and management (2004)
• Management of type 2 diabetes: BP and lipids (2002)

Blood glucose[£]: Aim to keep HbA$_{1c}$ <7.5%. If type 1 DM and high or moderately high risk of arterial disease, aim for HbA1c ≤6.5%.

BP[£]: Any ↓ in average BP ↓ risk of cardiovascular complications. Treat elevated BP ≥140/85 in all patients with DM with target BP of <130/80mmHg. Thiazides may be used as first line if no evidence of either microalbuminuria or albuminuria present when ACE inhibitors (or angiotensin receptor blocker) should be used as first line.

ⓘ Most diabetics will need combination therapy to achieve adequate control. Use ACE inhibitor as second line if thiazide diuretic used as first line or thiazide diuretic as second line of ACE inhibitor used as first line. Other suitable agents for use alone or in combination include β-blockers and alpha 2 receptor antagonists. Only use calcium-channel blockers as second-line or in combination therapy.

The diabetic foot: Foot problems are common amongst diabetics. 5% develop a foot ulcer in any year and amputation rates are 0.5%/y. Foot problems are due to:
● Peripheral neuropathy (affects 20–40% diabetic patients) → ↓ foot sensation *and*
● Peripheral vascular disease (affects 20–40% diabetic patients) → pain and predisposition to ulceration.

Risk factors
● Neuropathy
● Peripheral vascular disease
● Previous ulceration or amputation
● Age >70y.
● Plantar callus
● Foot deformities

● Poor footwear
● Long duration of DM
● Social deprivation and isolation
● Poor vision
● Smoking

Table 4.4 Clinical features of neuropathic and vascular foot ulcers	
Neuropathic	**Vascular**
Warm foot	Cool foot
Bounding pulses, normal ABI	Absent pulses, ↓ABI
Located at pressure points	Located at extremities (e.g. between toes)
Painless	Painful
Clearly defined or 'punched out'. Surrounded by callus	Less clearly delineated

ⓘ Diabetics may have coexisting peripheral neuropathy and peripheral vascular disease. ABI may be artificially ↑ due to calcification of vessels.

GMS contract			
DM 5	% of patients with DM who have a record of HbA₁c or equivalent in the 15mo.	up to 3 points	40–90%
DM 20	% of patients with DM with HbA₁c ≤7.5 (or equivalent test/reference range depending on local laboratory) in the previous 15mo.	up to 17 points	40–50%
DM 7	% of patients with DM with HbA₁c ≤10 (or equivalent test/reference range depending on local laboratory) in the previous 15mo.	up to 11 points	40–90%
DM 11	% of patients with DM who have a record of BP in the previous 15mo.	up to 3 points	40–90%
DM 12	% of patients with DM in whom the last BP is ≤145/85	up to 18 points	40–60%
DM 13	% of patients with DM who have a record of micro-albuminuria testing in the previous 15mo. (exception reporting if proteinuria)	up to 3 points	40–90%
DM 15	% of patients with DM with a diagnosis of proteinuria or micro-albuminuria who are treated with ACE inhibitors (or A2 antagonists)	up to 3 points	40–80%

Coronary heart disease: 📖 p.245
Hypertension: 📖 p.253

Advice for patients: Information and support

Diabetes UK ☎ 0845 120 2960 🖥 www.diabetes.org.uk

Further information
BS2 Joint British Societies guidelines on prevention of cardiovascular disease in clinical practice (2005). *Heart* 91 (Suppl. 5): v1-52
NICE 🖥 www.nice.org.uk
  Type 1 diabetes: diagnosis and management (2004)
  Type 2 diabetes: Prevention and management of foot problems (2004)

The diabetic foot check: Check the feet as part of annual review.

History
- Foot problems since last review
- Visual or mobility problems affecting self-care of feet
- Self-care behaviours and knowledge of foot care
- History of numbness, tingling or burning – may be worse at night

Examination
- Foot shape, deformity, joint rigidity and shoes
- Foot skin condition – fragility, cracking, oedema, callus, ulceration, sweating, presence of hair
- Foot and ankle pulses$^{£}$
- Sensitivity to 10g monofilament or vibration$^{£}$

Classification of foot risk: Table 4.5

Table 4.5 Classification of foot risk	
Foot risk	**Features**
Low current risk	Normal sensation, palpable pulses
Increased risk	Neuropathy, absent pulses or other risk factors
High risk	Neuropathy or absent pulses + deformity or skin changes or previous ulcer
Ulcerated foot	Foot ulcer on examination

Management
General points
- Optimize diabetic control and risk factors for vascular disease (including smoking cessation).
- Review drug therapy – stop β-blockers if evidence of peripheral vascular disease.
- Educate about foot care.

Specific management: Manage according to foot risk (Table 4.5).
- *Low risk:* Foot care education.
- *Increased risk:* Foot care education. Refer to the foot protection team. Check feet every 3–6mo. Consider referral for vascular assessment. Consider regular podiatry if poor vision, immobility or poor social conditions/foot hygiene. If previous foot ulcer, deformity or skin changes, manage as high risk.
- *High risk:* Stress importance of foot care. Refer to the foot protectio team for specialist podiatry. Inspect feet every 3–6mo. Review need for vascular assessment. Treat fungal infection.
- *Foot ulcer:* Refer to the multidisciplinary specialist foot care team urgently. Assess ischaemia using dopplers. Consider referral for angiography. Treat infection. If new ulceration, cellulitis or discolouration, refer to a specialised podiatry/foot care team within 24h.

GMS contract

DM 9	% of patients with diabetes with a record of presence or absence of peripheral pulses in the previous 15mo.	up to 3 points	40–90%
DM10	% of patients with diabetes with a record of neuropathy testing in the previous 15mo.	up to 3 points	40–90%

GP Notes:

What should diabetic patients do to look after their feet?
Advise patients to:
- Wash their feet daily and carefully dry them
- Check their feet daily looking for colour change, swelling, breaks in the skin and/or numbness
- Wear well-fitting shoes and hosiery
- Ensure their nails are cut regularly.

If patients are unable to check their feet themselves, explore ways to make this possible (e.g. use of mirrors) or make arrangements for regular checks by a chiropodist, district nurse or other healthcare professional.

🛈 Verruca or corn removal can be dangerous for diabetic patients as it can introduce infection into the foot. Advise patients to go to a chiropodist/podiatrist with experience in care of diabetic feet.

When should they seek help from a health professional?
- If there is any colour change of the feet, swelling, breaks in the skin or numbness *or*
- If self-monitoring is not possible (e.g. due to mobility problems).

Are there any additional precautions patients at increased or high risk of foot problems should take?
For patients at increased or high risk or with ulcers, additionally advise no barefoot walking and that, due to ↓ sensation, extra care and attention is needed.

If skin lesions advise patients to seek help if any change in the lesion, if ↑swelling, pain, odour, colour change or systemic symptoms.

167

Further information

NICE 🖳 www.nice.org.uk
- Type 1 diabetes: diagnosis and management (2004)
- Type 2 diabetes: prevention and management of foot problems (2004)

Hypertension

A major risk factor for coronary heart disease (CHD) and stroke (CVA), hypertension is underdiagnosed and undermanaged in the UK.

↑BP is symptomless until it causes organ damage. ~50% age 65–74y. have ↑BP. Management aims to detect and treat it before damage occurs.

Diagnosis of hypertension: BP is a continuous variable – the higher the BP, the greater the risk of CVA/CHD. There is no figure above which hypertension can be diagnosed definitively although currently treatment is considered at BP >140/90 (see Table 4.6, 🕮 p.171).

Isolated systolic hypertension[G]: Offer patients with isolated systolic hypertension (systolic BP >160mmHg) the same treatment as patients with both raised systolic and diastolic blood pressure.

Causes
- Unknown – 95% (essential hypertension) – alcohol (10%) or obesity may be contributory factors
- Renal disease
- Endocrine disease – Cushings (both syndrome and 2° to steroids), Conns syndrome, phaeochromocytoma, acromegaly, hyperparathyroidism, DM
- Pregnancy – 🕮 p.178
- Coarctation of the aorta – 🕮 p.118

Presentation
- Usually asymptomatic and found during routine BP screening or incidentally. Occasionally presents with headache or visual disturbance.
- End-organ damage – left ventricular hypertrophy, TIAs, previous stroke or myocardial infarct, angina, renal impairment, peripheral vascular disease, retinal vein occlusion.

Examination
- Check BP – 🕮 p.28
- Examine the heart – heart size, heart sounds, for heart failure
- Examine the fundi (Figure 4.3). *Eye signs include:*
    - Arteriolar vasoconstriction and arterio-venous 'nipping' – narrowing where vessels cross
    - Flame haemorrhages and/or hard exudates (Figure 4.4)
    - Retinal infarcts – cotton wool spots
    - Macular oedema and rarely papilloedema (associated with malignant hypertension)

🛈 BP varies throughout the day and can ↑ as a response to having BP checked ('white coat phenomenon' – prevalence 10%). Take ≥2 measurements on 2 occasions before classifying a patient as hypertensive.

Investigation
- *Blood:* FBC, U&E, creatinine, glucose, lipid profile, consider γGT if excess alcohol is a possibility
- *Urine:* RBCs, glucose, protein
- *ECG:* look for signs of left ventricular hypertrophy and ischaemia
- Consider *echo* if left ventricular hypertrophy is suspected

| Records 11 | BP of patients aged ≥45y. is recorded in the preceding 5y. for ≥65% of patients | 10 points |
| Records 17 | BP of patients aged ≥45y. is recorded in the preceding 5y. for ≥80% of patients | 5 points |

⚠ **Malignant hypertension:** *Presents with* headache, very elevated BP (diastolic >140mmHg), renal failure, fits, coma (encephalopathy) and severe retinopathy. Life-threatening condition. If malignant hypertension is suspected admit as an acute medical emergency.

Figure 4.3 Hypertensive retinopathy: arterial attenuation, exudates at the macula and haemorrhage

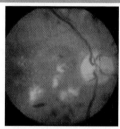

169

Figure 4.4 Macroaneurysm: haemorrhage and exudates around the inferior retinal artery

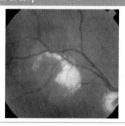

Figures 4.3 and 4.4 are reproduced from with permission from Southampton University Hospitals Trust.

Management of hypertension

Malignant hypertension: 📖 p.169

Aims
- Aim to ↓BP to <140/85 (diabetics, those with chronic renal failure or established atherosclerotic disease <130/80).
- Benefits of treatment remain in patients up to 85y. of age – and probably beyond. Offer patients >80y. the same treatment as young patients, taking into account any co-morbidity and existing drug use.

Non-drug treatment: Offer to all hypertensives and those with family history of ↑BP. Reinforce advice with written information.
- Offer smoking cessation advice and help[£] (📖 p.188).
- ↓ weight to optimum for height (📖 p.192).
- Encourage regular exercise – dynamic is best e.g. walking, swimming, cycling (📖 p.198).
- ↓ alcohol to <21u/wk. for ♂ and <14u/wk. for ♀ (📖 p.200).
- ↓ dietary salt intake.
- ↑ dietary fruit and vegetable intake – aim for 5 portions/d.
- ↓ excess coffee consumption and other caffeine-rich products.
- Encourage relaxation and stress management.
- *Don't* offer Ca^{2+}, Mg^{2+} or K^+ supplements as a method to ↓ BP.

Drug treatment
- *BP lowering drugs:* 📖 p.174
- *Aspirin* (📖 p.156): Recommend 75mg od for hypertensive patients if
  - aged ≥50y.
  - satisfactory control of BP (<150/90mmHg) *and*
  - target organ damage, DM or 10y. CVD risk ≥20%.
- *Statin therapy* (📖 p.182): Prescribe:
  - If ↑BP complicated by CVD irrespective of baseline cholesterol or LDL levels *or*
  - For 1° prevention in patients >40y. with ↑BP and 10y. CVD risk ≥20%.

Follow-up: Regular review of patients with ↑BP is essential. Once ↑BP is controlled, routine review of BP can be undertaken by properly trained practice nurses but annual review of medication should be undertaken by a GP and the GP must review if BP is not controlled.

Review interval: Depends on stability of BP:
- *After starting treatment:* Review after 1mo.
- *If BP is controlled:* Review after a further 3mo. and then every 3–6mo.
- *If BP is not controlled:*
  - Bring the patient back to repeat the BP reading. *Don't* alter medication on the strength of a single BP reading.
  - If ↑BP is sustained, alter medication – 📖 p.174. Most patients need >1 drug.
  - If ↑ dose causes ↑ side-effects without improvement in response, alter medication.
  - Review in the same way monthly until BP is controlled.

Table 4.6 Grades of hypertension and interventions

BP category	Systolic BP(mmHg)	Diastolic (mmHg)	Lifestyle intervention	Drug therapy
Normal	<120	<80	–	–
High nomal	135–9	85–9	Yes	Consider*
Mild hypertension (Grade 1)	140–159	90–99	Yes	Consider**
Moderate hypertension (Grade 2)	160–169	100–109	Yes	Yes
Severe hypertension (Grade 3)	≥180	≥110	Yes	Yes

*Drug treatment may be indicated for people with established cardiovascular disease, chronic renal disease or DM with complications

**Drug therapy is recommended for people with established cardiovascular disease, DM, target organ damage (heart failure, CHD, stroke/TIA, peripheral arterial disease. ↑ Cr, proteinuria/microalbuminuria, hypertension or diabetic retinopathy, left ventricular hypertrophy on Echo/ECG) or a 10y., CVD risk ≥20%

GMS contract: Hypertension management

BP 1	The practice can produce a register of patients with established hypertension	6 points	
BP 4	% of patients with hypertension in whom there is a record of BP in the past 9mo.	up to 20 points	40–90%
BP 5	% of patients with hypertension in whom the last BP (measured in the last 9mo.) is ≤150/90	up to 57 points	40–70%

GP Notes: Education

- Patients will not take tablets regularly, be motivated to change lifestyle or turn up for regular checks if they don't understand why treating ↑BP is important or side-effects they are likely to experience.
- On the other hand, some patients who were fit and well prior to their diagnosis assume a sick role unless it is explained that they are well and treatment is designed to stop illness developing.
- Reinforce management and give opportunities for discussion at every opportunity.

Table 4.6 is reproduced from JBS2: Joint British Societies' guidelines on prevention of cardiovascular disease in clinical practice. (2005). Heart 91 (Suppl. 5), with permission from BMJ Publishing Ltd.

Format of the annual review

- Check BP[£].
- Look for signs of end-organ failure—including annual urine test for proteinuria.
- Discuss symptoms and medication.
- Assess and treat other modifiable risk factors for CVD.
- Reinforce non-drug treatment (📖 p.170).

Referral to cardiology general medicine/renal physician

- Malignant hypertension (BP >180/110 + signs of papilloedema and/or retinal haemorrhage) or BP >220/110 – E
- Renal impairment (eGFR <60ml/min/1.73m^2 for >3mo., haematuria and/or proteinuria and UTI excluded) – U/S/R
- Suspected 2° hypertension – S/R
- Patients <35y. – R
- Multiple risk factors – R
- BP difficult to treat – R
- Pregnancy—to obstetrician—urgency depends on stage of pregnancy and clinical features – 📖 p.178

E = Emergency admission; U = Urgent; S = Soon; R = Routine

Reducing or stopping treatment: ↓BP too far (<120/80) may ↑ mortality – especially in the elderly.

- *Don't* stop medication if high CVD risk or end-organ damage.
- If diastolic BP <80 and systolic BP <140 consistently, consider decreasing or stopping medication. 1–2y. after withdrawal of medication 50% are normotensive and 40% stay off drug therapy permanently.
- Elderly people are prone to postural hypotension. Check for postural drop (sitting and standing BP). If present, ↓ dose of antihypertensive.
- Continue BP follow-up lifelong even if off medication.

172

Advice for patients: Information for patients and carers

British Heart Foundation ☎ 0845 0708 070 🖳 www.bhf.org.uk
Blood Pressure Association ☎ 020 8772 4994
🖳 www.bpassoc.org.uk

GMS contract: Hypertension and secondary prevention

Diabetes 11	% of patients with diabetes who have a record of BP in the prevous 15mo.	up to 3 points	40–90%
Diabetes 12	% of patients with diabetes in whom the last BP was ≤145/85	up to 18 points	40–60%
Stroke 5	% of patients with TIA/stroke who have a record of BP in the notes in the preceding 15mo.	up to 2 points	40–90%
Stroke 6	% of patients with a history of TIA/stroke in whom the last BP reading (measured in previous 15mo.) is ≤150/90	up to 5 points	40–70%
CHD 5	% of patients with coronary heart disease whose notes have a record of BP in the previous 15mo.	up to 7 points	40–90%
CHD 6	% of patients with coronary heart disease in whom the last BP reading (measured in the last 15mo.) is ≤150/90	up to 19 points	40–70%

GP Notes: Ways to improve concordance

- Discuss reasons for treatment and consequences of not treating the condition, ensuring information is tailored, clear, accurate, accessible and sufficiently detailed. Use simple language and avoid medical terms.
- Seek patients' views on their condition and agree the course of action before prescribing.
- Explain what the drug is, its function and (if known and not too complex) its mechanism of action.
- Keep the drug regime as simple as possible—od or bd dosing is preferable, especially long-term.
- Seek the patients, views on how they will manage the regime within their daily schedule and try to tie it in with daily routine (e.g. take one in the morning when you get up).
- Discuss possible side-effects, especially common or unpleasant side-effects.
- Give clear verbal instructions and reinforce with written instructions if it is a complex regime, the patient is elderly or understanding of the patient is in doubt.
- Deal with any questions the patient has and address further patient questions and practical difficulties at follow-up.
- Monitor repeat prescriptions.

urther information

NICE Hypertension – management of hypertension in adults in primary care (2004 and update 2006) ⌨ www.nice.org.uk

HS Guidelines for the management of hypertension (2004) www.bhsoc.org

BS2 Joint British Societies' guidelines on prevention of cardiovascular sease in clinical practice (2005). *Heart* **91** (suppl. 5): v1-52.

Drug treatment of hypertension

The 2 major guideline-producing bodies in the UK have now combined to produce consensus guidelines for the treatment of hypertension in primary care.

Recommendations for drug treatment Figure 4.5

> **General rules**
> - **If a drug is not tolerated:** Stop and move on to next line of therapy
> - **If a drug is tolerated but the BP target is not met:** Add in the next line of therapy.
> - **Where possible:** Recommend treatment with drugs taken only once a day and prescribe non-proprietary drugs which minimize cost.

≥55y. or black-skinned patients of African or Caribbean descent (an age): 1st choice intial therapy is a dihydropyridine calcium channel blocker (C) or thiazide-type diuretic (D).

Second line: if initial treatment was with a dihydropyridine calcium channel blocker or thiazide-type diuretic and a second drug is required add an ACE inhibitor (or angiotensin receptor blocker (ARB) if an ACE inhibitor is not tolerated).

<55y.: First-choice initial therapy is an ACE inhibitor (or ARB if the ACE inhibitor is not tolerated) (A).

Second line: If initial therapy was with an ACE inhibitor and a second drug is required, add a dihydropyridine calcium channel blocker or thiazide-type diuretic.

If treatment with 3 drugs is needed: Combine an ACE inhibitor, dihydropyridine calcium channel blocker and thiazide-type diuretic.

If treatment with 4 drugs is needed: Consider adding an alpha blocker or further diuretic therapy or a beta-blocker.

❗ If blood pressure remains uncontrolled with the addition of a 4 drug, refer for specialist advice.

Beta blockers: β-blockers are no longer recommended as a routine initial therapy for hypertension.

Exceptions: β-blockers may be considered as a first line treatment of:
- younger women of child-bearing potential or
- patients with hypertension and evidence of ↑ sympathetic drive or
- patients intolerant of or with contraindications to ACE inhibitors/ARBs

In these circumstances, if initial therapy is with a β-blocker and a 2 drug is required, add a dihydropyridine calicum-channel blocker.

Patients already on β-blockers: If a patient's blood pressure is well controlled on a β-blocker there is no need to change it. If not controlled, change treatment according to the new recommendation Gradually step down dose of β-blockers when withdrawing them.

⚠ Do NOT withdraw β-blockers in patients with other good reason to take them e.g. angina or post-MI.

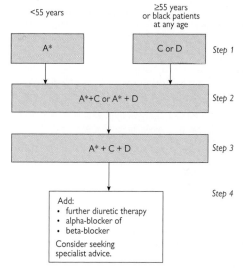

Figure 4.5 Algorithm for drug treatment of newly diagnosed hypertension

<55 years

≥55 years or black patients at any age

| A* | C or D | Step 1 |

A*+C or A* + D — Step 2

A* + C + D — Step 3

Step 4

Add:
- further diuretic therapy
- alpha-blocker of
- beta-blocker

Consider seeking specialist advice.

A = ACE inhibitor (* or ARB if ACE inhibitor is not tolerated)
C = Calcium channel blocker
D = Thiazide diuretic

🛈 In the absence of other evidence, black-skinned patients *not* of African or Caribbean descent, should be treated according to the algorithm as non-black.

ʒure 4.5 is reproduced with permission from NICE Hypertension: Management of hypertenɔn in adults in primary care: partial update (2006). CG34. www.nice.org.uk

Table 4.7 First-line antihypertensive drugs

Class of 1st line drug	Reasons to choose the drug	Reasons to avoid the drug
α-blockers BNF 2.5.4	Prostatism Dyslipidaemia	Urinary incontinence worsens. Postural hypotension is common.
ACE inhibitors BNF 2.5.5.1 ❗ Check U&E and Cr before starting and at first follow-up.	Heart failure or left ventricular dysfunction Post-MI or established CVD Diabetic nephropathy 2° stroke prevention	*Do not use:* If known renovascular disease – can precipitate renal failure, or in pregnancy.
Angiotensin receptor blocker (ARB) BNF 2.5.5.2 ❗ Check U&E and Cr before starting and monitor K^+ at follow-up.	ACE inhibitor intolerance Diabetic nephropathy ↑BP + LVH Heart failure if ACE intolerant Post-MI	*Use with caution:* If aortic or mitral valve stenosis and in obstructive hypertrophic cardiomyopathy
β-blockers BNF 2.4 ❗ May accumulate in patients with renal failure – ↓ dose.	No longer recommended as a first line drug for hypertension	*Avoid in patients with:* Asthma, COPD, heart block, heart failure, peripheral vascular disease, hyperlipidaemia. *In patients with DM:* May → small deterioration in glucose tolerance and ↓ awareness of hypoglycaemia.
Calcium-channel blockers BNF 2.6.2 ❗ Different agents have different therapeutic effects.	*Dihydropyridine agents:* Of proven efficacy in the elderly and those with isolated systolic hypertension. *Rate-limiting agents:* Useful in those with angina or post-MI.	*Rate-limiting agents:* Avoid in patients with heart block or heart failure. Do not combine with β-blockers.
Thiazide diuretics BNF 2.2.1 ❗ Use the lowest dose. Higher doses don't have additional effect on BP.	More effective than β-blockers in the elderly.	Avoid in patients with gout. May adversely affect lipid profile and blood glucose.
❗ Most patients require >1 drug to control their BP.		
⚠ Avoid combination of β-blockers and rate-limiting calcium antagonists (verapamil, diltiazem) due to risk of bradycardia/asystole.		

Advice for patients: Patient experiences of high blood pressure

Discovery

'I went to visit my GP...amongst other things, he took my blood pressure and noted that it was quite high...Then I was invited to come in again, I think the following week, and they checked my blood pressure a number of times.'

'There was this stand where they had these automatic blood pressure measuring machines, where the machine sort of pumps up your blood pressure and measures it. So I thought "Oh well, it's fun, I'll just try this out." And I tried it out and it was something absolutely appalling, like 180 over 120.'

Medication

'I had a number of alternatives...I could lose weight, I could try and give up salt, I could take lots of exercise and see if that had any effect on my blood pressure. And, yes, I tried those...It finally became obvious that I would need to go on tablets.'

'Apparently medication will bring the blood pressure down, undoubtedly it will – but who knows what else it's doing to you, that's what I always feel...But if it stops me having a stroke or a heart attack then obviously I've got to take it.'

'Sometimes I'm a bit worried because sometimes I experience dizziness; sometimes I feel a bit lethargic and just feel peculiar. In the first instance I thought, well, maybe it was me. Then I began to think I'm taking all these medications...they must have some effect so it might be because of those medications.'

'Well there are two factors affecting my pill taking in this area. I am extremely forgetful...I just lead a very busy life and one just forgets. But there is a factor that every time one takes the pill it reminds one that one is less than perfect. One has hypertension and I hate that.'

'I very, very occasionally forget to take my medication as it tends to be built into my daily routine. I'm sure everybody does this: get up, go and get the water, take them. But very occasionally, say if something wakes you like a phone call and you're not treading the same little path that you always tread to the tap and then back to the tablets, if something breaks then you might forget.'

Hypertension in pregnancy

Chronic hypertension or essential hypertension: Present before or <20wk into pregnancy. More common in older mothers and there may be a FH. Chronic hypertension may worsen in later pregnancy. Consider changing medication to drugs known to be safe in pregnancy pre-conceptually or as soon as pregnancy is confirmed (Table 4.8). Aim to keep BP <140/90. Risk of pre-eclampsia is ↑ ×5 (see below).

Pregnancy-induced hypertension (PIH): ↑ BP appearing >20wk into pregnancy and resolving <3mo. after delivery. Affects 10% of pregnancies and risk of pre-eclampsia is ↑. Treatment is the same as for chronic hypertension. ↑ risk of developing hypertension later in life.

Pre-eclampsia^G *(pregnancy induced hypertension and proteinuria or pre eclamptic toxaemia (PET))*: Affects 5–7% of primigravida and 2–3% of all pregnancies. Multisystem disease of unknown cause, developing ≥20wk into pregnancy and only resolving once the baby is delivered (<10d. after birth). Risk factors – Box 4.1. Untreated, may progress to eclampsia – the most common cause of death from pregnancy in the UK.

Criteria for diagnosis
● BP >140/90 or >+30/+15 from booking The earlier in pregnancy the BP rises, the more likely the pre-eclampsia will be severe.
● Proteinuria ≥0.3/24h. – urine dipstick is a useful screening tool – if ≥1+ protein then probably significant – but ~25% false +ve rate

⚠ Pre-eclampsia is asymptomatic until its terminal phase, and onset may be rapid, so frequent BP screening is essential. Whenever you check BP in pregnancy, always check urine for protein

Interval for routine BP checks
● If no risk factors for pre-eclampsia (Box 5.7) – routine antenatal care
● If 1 risk factor for pre-eclampsia but no factor which requires referral in early pregnancy, from 24–32wk. gestation, re-check BP at least every 3wk., and >32wk. gestation, re-check at least every 2wk.
● If >1 risk factor or factor which requires referral in early pregnancy, refer <20 wk. and then monitor as directed by the specialist.

Thresholds for further action: Table 4.9, 📖 p.180

Prevention
● Low-dose aspirin may benefit for high-risk, women (i.e those who have a past history of pre-eclampsia) – refer for advice.
● Other possible interventions (ongoing trials): rest, calcium supplements if low dietary calcium, antioxidants (especially Vitamins C and E)

Risk of recurrence
● Risk of recurrence in subsequent pregnancy with the same partner is 10–15% but usually less severe.
● Women who have pre-eclampsia are at greater risk of developing ↑ BP later in life.

Table 4.8 Drugs for hypertension which are safe in pregnancy	
Drug	**Notes**
Methyldopa	First choice. Doses <1g/d. cause less drowsiness
β-blockers	e.g. labetolol. Use with caution, preferably only the 3rd trimester
Nifedipine	Modified release preparations (unlicensed). Manufacturer advises use with caution
α-blocker	e.g. doxazosin, Manufacturer advises use with caution

Box 4.1 Risk factors for pre-eclampsia – evaluate at booking[G]

Refer early (<20 wk.) for specialist care if
- Pre-eclampsia/eclampsia in previous pregnancy
- Multiple pregnancy
- Underlying medical conditions:
  - Pre-existing hypertension or booking diastolic BP ≥90mmHg
  - Pre-existing renal disease or booking proteinuria ≥1 + on >1 occasion or quanified as ≥0.3g/24h.
  - Pre-existing DM
  - Antiphospholipid antibodies
- ≥2 other risk factors:
  - First pregnancy (or first time by a new partner)
  - Age ≥40y.
  - BMI ≥35 or <18kg/m^2
  - Family history of eclampsia/ pre-eclampsia (particularly mother/sister)
  - Booking diastolic BP ≥80 but <90mmHg

179

⚠ Significant symptons/signs of pre-eclampsia

- New hypertension
- New and/or significant proteinuria
- Maternal symptoms of headache and/or visual disturbance
- Maternal epigastric pain and/or vomiting
- Reduced foetal movements or small for gestational age infant

HELLP syndrome: occurs in pregnancy or <48h. after delivery Associated with severe pre-eclampsia.
- **H**aemolysis
- **E**levated **L**iver enzymes
- **L**ow **P**latelets

Signs
- Hypertension (80%)
- Right upper quadrant pain (90%)
- Nausea and vomiting (50%)
- Oedema

Management: Admit as for pre-eclampsia (opposite)

Table 4.9 Thresholds for further action

Findings (BP readings are in mmHg)		Action
New hypertension without proteinuria >20wk. gestation	Diastolic BP ≥90 and <100mmHg	Refer for specialist assessment* in <48h
	Diastolic BP ≥90 and <100mmHg with significant symptoms (below)	Refer for same day specialist assessment*
	Diastolic BP ≥100mmHg	
	Systolic BP ≥160mmHg	
New hypertension without proteinuria >20wk. gestation	Diastolic BP ≥90 and new proteinuria ≥1+ on dipstick	Refer for same day specialist assessment*
	Diastolic BP ≥90 and new proteinuria ≥1+ on dipstick and significant symptoms (below)	Immediate admission
	Diastolic BP ≥110 and new proteinuria ≥1+ on dipstick	
	Systolic BP ≥170 and new proteinuria ≥1+ on dipstick	
New proteinuria without hypertension >20wk. gestation	1+ on dipstick	Repeat pre-eclampsia assessment in <1wk
	2+ on dipstick	Refer for specialist assessment* in <48h
	≥1+ on dipstick with significant symptoms (below)	Refer for same day specialist assessment*
Maternal symptoms or foetal signs/ symptoms without new hypertension or proteinuria	Headache and/or visual disturbance with diastolic BP <90 and trace or no proteinuria	Investigate cause of headache. ↓ interval to next pre-eclampsia assessment
	Epigastric pain with diastolic BP <90 and trace or no proteinuria	If simple antacids are ineffective, refer for same day specialist assessment*
	↓ foetal movements or small for gestational age infant with diastolic BP <90 and trace or no proteinuria	Refer for investigation of foetal compromise. ↓ interval to next pre-eclampsia assessment

⚠ Significant symptoms

- Epigastic pain
- Vomiting
- Headache
- Visual disturbance
- ↓ foetal movements
- Small for gestational age infant

*Most obstetric departments have a day case 'step-up' assessment unit

Further information

APEC Pre-eclampsia community guideline (2004) ⌨ www.apec.org.uk
RCOG Pre-eclampsia- study group recommendations (2003)
⌨ www.rcog.org.uk

Table 4.9 is reproduced with permission from APEC, ⌨ www.apec.org.uk

Advice for patients: Frequently asked questions about pre-eclampsia

What is eclampsia and pre-eclampsia? Pre-eclampsia usually only occurs after the 20th week of pregnancy. It causes high blood pressure and protein to leak into the urine. Eclampsia may follow on from pre-eclampsia (1 in 100 women with pre-eclampsia). It is a type of fit (or seizure) which is a life-threatening complication of pregnancy.

Why have I got pre-eclampsia? Any pregnant women can develop pre-eclampsia (1 in 14 pregnancies). You have increased risk if you;
● Are pregnant for the first time (1 in 30 women get pre-eclampsia), or are pregnant for the first time by a new partner.
● Have had pre-eclampsia before.
● Have a family history of pre-eclampsia. Particulary if it occurred in your mother or sister.
● Had high blood pressure before the pregnancy started.
● Are diabetic, or have systemic lupus erythematosis (SLE) or chronic kidney disease.
● Are aged below 20 or above 35.
● Have a pregnancy with twins, triplets, or more.
● Are obese.

What causes pre-eclampsia? No-one really knows. It is probably due to a problem with the placenta (the afterbirth).

How do you know I have pre-eclampsia? Most women do not feel ill or have any symptoms at first. Pre-eclampsia is present if:
● your blood pressure becomes high, *and*
● you have an abnormal amount of protein in your urine.

Severity of pre-eclampsia is usually (but not always) related to the blood pressure level. Other symptoms which suggest severe pre-eclampsia are:
● Headaches
● Blurring of vision, or other visual problems
● Abdominal (tummy) pain – usually just below the ribs
● Vomiting
● Just not feeling right

Swelling or puffiness of your feet, face, or hands (oedema) is also a feature of pre-eclampsia but is also common in normal pregnancy.

How is pre-eclampsia treated? Regular checks may be all that you need if pre-eclampsia remains relatively mild. If pre-eclampsia becomes worse, you are likely to be admitted to hospital. Tests may be done to check on your well-being, and that of your baby. As the only way of stopping the pre-eclampsia is to deliver the baby, in some cases babies are delivered early to prevent harm to mother or baby.

Will pre-eclampsia develop in my next pregnancy? If you had pre-eclampsia in your first pregnancy, you have about a 1 in 10 chance of it recurring in future pregnancies.

Further information

Action on pre-EClampsia (APEC) ☎ 020 8863 3271
🖥 www.apec.org.uk

Hyperlipidaemia

Average cholesterol level in a population is a predictor of CVD risk and dependent on diet but, on an individual level, it is a much poorer predictor – only 42% who develop CHD have ↑ cholesterol. However, lowering cholesterol is of proven benefit in 1° and 2° prevention of CVD. Concern that low cholesterol is associated with ↑ risk of death from other causes (e.g. suicide, cancer) is unfounded.

Cholesterol: Fatty substance manufactured by the body (mainly liver) which plays a vital role in functioning of cell membranes. Total plasma cholesterol consists of:

- **LDL (low density lipoprotein) cholesterol** – high levels associated with ↑ risk CVD
- **HDL (high density lipoprotein) cholesterol** – low levels associated with ↑ risk CVD
- **Triglycerides (TGs)** – independent risk factor for CVD. If >5mmol/l refer for specialist opinion.
- **Ratio of total cholesterol:HDL** – used to predict risk. No threshold – the higher the ratio, the greater the risk.

Testing for hyperlipidaemia: Blood cholesterol concentration is not steady over time. 1:4 ↑ cholesterols are normal on repeat testing. Check ≥2 samples at different times:

- **Before initiating treatment or if screening for familial dyslipidaemia** – take fasting samples checking triglycerides.
- **Screening and routine follow-up** – take non-fasting samples testing total blood cholesterol and total cholesterol:HDL ratio.

Screening

1° prevention: Opportunistically screen all adults ≥40y. for CVD risk even if no personal or family history of CVD or DM. Risk assessment should include:

- Ethnicity
- Smoking habit
- Family history of CVD
- Measurement of weight, waist circumference and BP
- Blood for non-fasting lipids (total cholesterol + HDL cholesterol) and non-fasting glucose

Total CVD risk can then be estimated using charts (Figures 4.1 and 4.2 📖 p.154–5). If risk ≥20% over 10y. intervention with lifestyle and/or drug measures to ↓ risk is justified.

2° prevention: All those who have proven CVD – check cholesterol levels annually.

Familial hyperlipidaemia: Screen 1st degree blood relatives >18y. old with fasting lipids if:

- FH of familial hyperlipidaemia
- FH of premature CHD (men <55y., women <65y.) or other atherosclerotic disease.
  Screening interval has not been determined – 5y. seems reasonable.

GMS contract			
DM 16	% of patients with diabetes who have a record of total cholesterol in the previous 15mo.	up to 3 points	40–90%
DM 17	% of patients with diabetes whose last measured total cholesterol within the previous 15mo. was ≤5mmol/l	up to 6 points	40–70%
Stroke 7	% of patients with TIA/stroke who have a record of total cholesterol in the previous 15mo.	up to 2 points	40–90%
Stroke 8	% of patients with TIA/stroke whose last measured total cholesterol (measured in previous 15mo.) was ≤5mmol/l	up to 5 points	40–60%
CHD 7	% of patients with coronary heart disease whose notes have a record of total cholesterol in the previous 15mo.	7 points	40–90%
CHD 8	% of patients with coronary heart disease whose last measured total cholesterol (measured in the previous 15mo.) is ≤5mmol/l	17 points	40–70%

Familial hyperlipidaemia: There are many types of familial dyslipidaemia. If suspected, refer. Common forms include:

- *Polygenic hypercholesterolaemia:* Most common form of familial dyslipidaemia. Presents with FH of premature CHD + ↑ total cholesterol.
- *Familial combined hyperlipidaemia:* Polygenic hyperlipidaemia affecting 0.5–1% of the population and ~15% of those suffering MI <60y. Associated with obesity, insulin resistance/DM, ↑BP, xanthelasma, corneal arcus and premature IHD. ↑ total cholesterol (6.5–10mmol/l); ↑ TGs (2.3–12mmol/l).
- *Familial hypercholesterolaemia* (type IIa): Autosomal dominant. Heterozygous form present in 1:500. Associated with tendon xanthomata and FH premature IHD. ↑ LDL (>4.9mmol/l); ↑ total cholesterol (>7.5mmol/l); normal TGs.
- *Familial hypertriglyceridaemia* (type IV/V): Autosomal dominant. Affects ~1% of the general population and ~5% having MI <60y. Associated with DM, obesity, gout, eruptive xanthomas and pancreatitis. Normal (or slightly ↑) total cholesterol; ↑ TGs (2.3–>10mmol/l).

Secondary hyperlipidaemia: Conditions associated with 2° hyperlipidaemia include:

- Drugs:
  - Steroids
  - β-blockers
  - Thiazides
  - COC pill
  - Isotretinoin
- Obesity
- DM
- Excess alcohol
- Pregnancy
- Hypothyroidism*
- Renal failure
- Nephrotic syndrome
- Cholestasis
- Cushing's syndrome
- Porphyria
- Myeloma
- Lipodystrophies
- Glycogen storage disease

* Patients with hypothyroidism should receive adequate thyroid replacement before assessing need for lipid-lowering treatment. Correction of hypothyroidism may resolve the lipid abnormality and untreated hypothyroidism ↑ risk of myositis with statins.

Management of hypercholesterolaemia: 📖 p.186

Advice for patients: Information for patients and carers

British Heart Foundation ☎ 0845 0708 070 🖥 www.bhf.org.uk

Further information

JBS2 Joint British Societies' Guidelines on prevention of Cardiovascular disease in clinical practice (2005). *Heart* **91** (suppl. 5): v1–52

NICE ▢ www.nice.org.uk

- Statins for the prevention of cardiovascular events in patients at increased risk of developing cardiovascular disease or those with established cardiovascular disease (2006)
- Cardiovascular risk assessment: the modification of blood lipids for the primary and secondary prevention of cardiovascular disease (due for publication in December 2007)

Lancet MRC/BHF *Heart Protection Study of cholesterol lowering with simvastatin of 5963 people with diabetes: a randomized placebo-controlled trial* (2003) **362** p. 2005–2016

Lancet 4S Group. *Randomised trial of cholesterol lowering in 4444 patients with coronary heart disease: the Scandinavian simvastatin survival study (4S)* (1994) **344** p. 1383–1389

NEJM Shepherd *et al.* *Prevention of coronary heart disease with pravastatin in men with hypercholesterolaemia* (1995) **333** p. 1301–1306

JAMA Schwartz *et al.* *Effects of atorvastatin on early recurrent ischaemic events in acute coronary syndromes: the miracle study: a randomised controlled trial* (2001) **285** p. 1771–1781

Lancet Sever *et al.* *Prevention of coronary and stroke events with atorvastatin in hypertensive patients who have average or lower than average cholesterol concentrations, in the Anglo Scandinavian cardiac outcomes trial lipid-lowering Harman (ASCOT-LLA): a multicentre randomised controlled trial* (2003) **361** p. 1149–1158

Journal of Human Hypertension The BHS Guidelines Working Party Guidelines for management of hypertension: report of the fourth working party of the British Hypertension Society (2004) **18** p. 138–185

Management of hypercholesterolaemia

Lowering LDL and raising HDL ↓ progression of coronary atherosclerosis – whatever the age of the patient.

Calculating cardiovascular disease (CVD) risk: Always consider ↑ cholesterol with other risk factors for CHD/CVD. Calculate risk using tables – 📖 p.154–5 – or a computer program e.g. Joint British Societies' Cardiac Risk Assessor (available free at 🖥 www. bhsoc.org).

ℹ Decisions on whether to treat ↑ cholesterol have been based in recent years on CHD risk but this should now be changed to CVD risk to reflect the importance of stroke as well as CHD prevention.

Non-drug therapy: Offer to all patients with ↑ cholesterol and those with DM or FH of CHD/CVD. Reinforce advice with written information.

- Decrease dietary fat to ≤30% of total energy intake
- Decrease saturated fat to ≤10% of total fat intake
- Decrease dietary cholesterol to <300mg/d
- Margarines and other foods enriched with plant sterol or stanol esters inhibit cholesterol absorption from the GI tract and can ↓ serum cholesterol in those on an average diet by 10%. Their effect on individuals already on a low fat diet is less.
- Weight ↓ – in patients with BMI ≥30kg/m², weight ↓ of 10kg → 7% ↓ in LDL and 13% ↑ in HDL.
- ↑ physical activity – enhances cholesterol-lowering effects of diet and weight ↓.
- Give general advice about ↓ CHD/CVD risk e.g. smoking cessation.

Drug therapy with statins

1° prevention

- **10y. CVD risk ≥20%** – initiate statin if total cholesterol >4mmol/l or LDL cholesterol >2mmol/l. Reducing cholesterol reduces all causes of mortality by 22% and ↓ CHD events by 31%.
- **DM** – initiate statin if ≥40y., or age 18–39y. and ≥1 of:
  - retinopathy
  - nephropathy
  - poor glycaemic control
  - ↑ BP requiring treatment
  - ↑ cholesterol ≥6mmol/l
  - features of metabolic syndrome
  - family history of premature CVD in a first degree relative.

2° prevention: Although statin treatment is often only offered to patients with total cholesterol >5mmol/l at present, trial data suggest *all* patients with proven CHD benefit from ↓ in total cholesterol and LDL irrespective of initial cholesterol concentration[S]. ↓ in total cholesterol and LDL by 25–35% using statin therapy → ↓ CHD mortality by 25–35%[S].

Treatment target[G]: Aim to ↓ total cholesterol by 25% or to <4mmol/l – whichever is the lower value, *or* to ↓ LDL cholesterol by 30% or to <2.0mmol/l – whichever is the lower value. LDL cholesterol levels are most important in ↓ CV risk.

Minimum audit standard[G]: Total cholesterol <5.0mmol/l or LDL cholesterol <3.0mmol/l or ↓ by 25% or 30%, respectively – whichever is the lower value. All type 2 diabetics offered a statin.

Referral to cardiology/general medicine: R = routine
- Familial hypercholesterolaemia (± referral to genetics) – R
- High triglycerides – R
- Hypercholesterolaemia resistant to treatment or difficult to treat – R

GP Notes: Frequently asked questions about statins

Which statin is best?
There is evidence from randomized controlled trials of efficacy of simvastatin and pravastatin. Other statins e.g. fluvastatin or atorvastatin may be cheaper.

What dose should I use?
Base the dose either on doses used in trials (simvastatin 20mg/ pravastatin 40mg) or start at the lowest dose, measure cholesterol 4–6 weekly, and titrate the dose upwards until target levels are reached.

Statins are most effective taken in the evening.

Are there any adverse effects I should warn patients about?
The most important adverse effect is myositis (<1:10,000). Ask patients to report any unexplained muscle pain/weakness. If this occurs check creatinine kinase – if >5x upper limit of normal, withdraw therapy.

What are the contraindications to statin use?
Pregnancy, breast-feeding and active liver disease are all contraindications to prescribing statins.

Are there any important interactions I should consider?
Statins ↑ the effect of warfarin.

The risk of myositis is ↑ when taken with other lipid-lowering drugs, macrolide antibiotics (e.g. erythromycin) or ciclosporin.

How should I monitor statin use?
- Take a fasting blood sample for cholesterol, triglycerides and glucose pre-treatment.
- Measure total cholesterol (non-fasting) 4–6wk. after starting treatment or after any dose change. If stable measure 6–12 monthly.
- Measure liver function tests pre-treatment and after 1–3mo. Thereafter measure each 6mo. for 1y. Discontinue if serum transaminase ↑ (and stays at) >3x normal.

What should I do if a patient is intolerant to statins?
Intolerance to statins is uncommon (<2% of patients). Use of other drugs (e.g. fibrates) is an alternative, either alone or in combination with low-dose statins.

Smoking

Facts and figures

- In the UK, 12 million adults (28% ♂; 26% ♀) smoke cigarettes and a further 3 million smoke pipes or cigars.
- Prevalence is highest in the 20–24y. old age group.
- 1% school children are smokers when they enter secondary school; by 15y., 22% are smoking.
- 82% of smokers start as teenagers.
- Government targets aim to ↓ smoking to ≤24% by 2010, and ↓ smoking amongst children to ≤9% by 2010.
- Surveys of smokers show 70% want to stop and 30% intend to give up in <1y. – but only ~2%/y. successfully give up permanently.

Risks of smoking: Smoking is the greatest single cause of illness and premature death in the UK. ½ all regular smokers will eventually die as a result of smoking – 120,000 people/y.

Tobacco smoking is associated with ↑ risk of

- *Cancers:* lung (>90% are smokers); lip; mouth; stomach; colon; bladder ~30% ALL cancer deaths
- *Cardiovascular disease:* arteriosclerosis, coronary heart disease, stroke, peripheral vascular disease
- *DM*
- *Chronic lung disease:* COPD, recurrent chest infection, exacerbation of asthma
- *Dyspepsia and/or gastric ulcers*
- *Thrombosis* (especially if also on the COC pill)
- *Osteoporosis*
- *Problems in pregnancy:* PET, IUGR, pre-term delivery, neonatal & late fetal death.

Passive smoking is associated with

- ↑ risk CHD & lung cancer (↑ by 25%)
- ↑ risk of cot death, bronchitis and otitis media in children.

Nicotine withdrawal symptoms

- Urges to smoke (70%)
- ↑ appetite (70% – average 3–4kg weight gain)
- Depression (60%)
- Restlessness (60%)
- Poor concentration (60%)
- Irritability/aggression (50%)
- Night-time awakenings (25%)
- Light-headedness (usually 1st few days after quitting – 10%)

Helping people to stop smoking: Advice from a GP about smoking cessation results in 2% of smokers stopping – 5% if advice is repeated[CE]. Strong motivation (often 2° to an episode of poor health directly related to smoking e.g. MI) is a vital factor.

GMS contract: Primary prevention

Records 22	% of patients aged >15y. whose notes record smoking status in the past 27mo. except for those who have never smoked where smoking status need be recorded only once	up to 11 points	40–90%
Information 5	The practice supports smokers in stopping smoking by a strategy which includes providing literature and offering appropriate therapy	2 points	

Advice for patients: A patient's experience of stopping smoking

'Although for several years previous to it [a heart attack] I had more than halved my consumption to 20 or so a day. Well, a week in hospital without so much as a crafty drag was a good start. Thereafter I just put cigarettes out of my mind.'

'Despite what is said about the powerful addictive nature of nicotine, if you have a strong enough motivation then giving up smoking is not at all difficult. If on the other hand you are applying will-power to something you don't really wish to succeed at, then neither chewing gum, patches nor hypnotism are going to be much help.'

'In my case the motivation was the threat to physical activity. I've never been remotely athletic, or a regular player of sport, but I do like walking and I positively seem to need the more active aspects of gardening and DIY. The immediate consequence of a heart attack made me realise how much I prized this sense of physical freedom and how much it was threatened. On that basis anything that might restrict or delay recovery was automatically out, and smoking was the most prominent candidate.'

Useful contacts for patients
Action on Smoking and Health (ASH) ☎ 020 7739 5902 🖳 www.ash.org.uk
NHS smoking helpline ☎ 0800 169 0 169; pregnancy smoking helpline ☎ 0800 169 9 169 🖳 www.gosmokefree.co.uk
Quit Helpline ☎ 0800 00 22 00 🖳 www.quit.org.uk

189

Further information
Clinical Evidence *Cardiovascular disorders: changing behaviour – smoking cessation* 🖳 www.library.nhs.uk
NICE Nicotine replacement therapy and bupropion for smoking cessation (2002) 🖳 www.nice.org.uk
Nicotine replacement therapy and buproprion for smoking cessation (2002)
Brief interventions and referral for smoking cessation in primary care and other settings (2006)
Cochrane Silagy C et al. *Nicotine replacement for smoking cessation* (2004) 🖳 www.library.nhs.uk

Aids to smoking cessation: *BNF 4.10*

Nicotine replacement therapy (NRT)
- ↑ the chance of stopping ~1½ x[N].
- All preparations are equally effective[C] and available on NHS prescription.
- Start with higher doses for patients highly dependent.
- Continue treatment for 3mo., tailing off dose gradually over 2wk. before stopping (except gum which can be stopped abruptly).
- Several preparations are now licensed for use in pregnancy if unable to stop without NRT.
- Contraindicated immediately post MI, stroke or TIA, and for patients with arrhythmia.

Bupropion (Zyban™)
- Smokers (>18y.) start taking the tablets 1–2wk. before their intended quit day (150mg od for 3d. then 150mg bd for 7–9wk.).
- ↑ cessation rate >2x[N].
- *Contraindications:* epilepsy or ↑ risk of seizures, eating disorder, bipolar disorder, pregnancy/breast-feeding.

Alternative therapies: There is some evidence hypnotherapy is helpful in some cases[S].

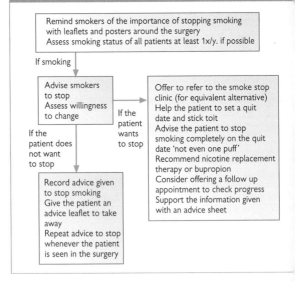

Figure 4.6 Management plan for smokers in the surgery

Remind smokers of the importance of stopping smoking with leaflets and posters around the surgery
Assess smoking status of all patients at least 1x/y. if possible

If smoking

Advise smokers to stop
Assess willingness to change

If the patient does not want to stop

If the patient wants to stop

Record advice given to stop smoking
Give the patient an advice leaflet to take away
Repeat advice to stop whenever the patient is seen in the surgery

Offer to refer to the smoke stop clinic (for equivalent alternative)
Help the patient to set a quit date and stick to it
Advise the patient to stop smoking completely on the quit date 'not even one puff'
Recommend nicotine replacement therapy or bupropion
Consider offering a follow up appointment to check progress
Support the information given with an advice sheet

Smoking 1	% of patients with any, or any combination of the following conditions: • coronary heart disease • DM • stroke or TIA • COPD *or* • hypertension • asthma whose notes record smoking status in the previous 15mo. Except those who have never smoked where smoking status need only be recorded once since diagnosis	up to 33 points	40–90%
Smoking 2	% of patients with any, or any combination of the conditions listed in 'Smoking 1' whose notes contain a record that smoking cessation advice or referral to a specialist service, where available, has been offered within the previous 15mo.	up to 35 points	40–90%

GP Notes:

⚠ Prescibe *only* for smokers who commit to target stop date. Initially prescribe only enough to last 2wk. after the target stop date i.e 2wk. nicotine replacement therapy or 3–4wk. bupropion. Only offer a 2nd prescription if the smoker demonstrates continuing commitment to stop smoking.

🕐 If unsuccessful the NHS will not fund another attempt for ≥6mo.

Obesity

Obesity is one of the most important preventable diseases in the UK. The best measure of obesity is body mass index (BMI). Recent evidence shows it is increasing and is set to take over from smoking as the number one preventable cause of disease in the UK.

Classification: BMI (weight in kg ÷ (height in m)^2):
- 18.5–24.9 normal
- 25–29.9 overweight
- 30–39.9 obese
- >40 morbid obesity

Health risks of obesity
- Death (BMI >30 carries 3x ↑ risk of mortality)
- IHD
- Hypercholesterolaemia
- ↑BP
- Cerebrovascular disease
- Type 2 DM
- Gallbladder disease
- Complications after surgery
- Sleep apnoea
- Psychological problems
- Cancer of cervix, uterus, ovary and breast
- Musculoskeletal problems and arthritis
- Ovulatory failure
- Menstrual irregularities
- Polycystic ovaries syndrome
- Complications in pregnancy (gestational DM, ↑BP, pre-eclampsia), labour and delivery
- Stress incontinence

Waist circumference: An alternative indirect measurement of body fat that reflects the intra-abdominal fat mass. Strongly correlated with CHD risk, DM, hyperlipidaemia and ↑BP (Table 4.10). Measure halfway between the superior iliac crest and the rib cage in the mid axillary line.

Risk factors
- Genetic predisposition (accounts for about $^1/_3$ obesity)
- Previous obesity and successful dieting
- Physical inactivity
- Low education
- Smoking cessation
- Female gender

Prevention: Begins in childhood by instilling healthy patterns of exercise and diet.

❶ There is little evidence to show that dietary advice by GPs or practice nurses is heeded. Most influence on diet comes from national food policy, price of food, advertising, general education and cultural influences.

GMS contract			
Obesity 1	The practice can produce a register of patients aged ≥16y. with a BMI ≥30 in the last 15mo.	8 points	
Diabetes 2	% of patients with diabetes whose notes record body mass index in the previous 15mo.	up to 3 points	40–90%

Table 4.10 Association of waist circumference with risk of CHD and DM

	Waist circumference	
	White Caucasians	*Asians*
♂	≥102cm (40 inches)	≥90cm (36 inches)
♀	≥88cm (35 inches)	≥80cm (32 inches)

Further information

National Audit Office *Tackling obesity in England* (2001)
 www.nao.org.uk
NICE www.nice.org.uk
  Obesity: the prevention, identification, assessment and management of overweight and obesity in adults and children (2006)
  Guidance on the use of sibutramine for the treatment of obesity in adults (2001)
  Orlistat for treatment of obesity in adults (2001)
National Obesity Forum www.nationalobesityforum.org.uk
  Guidelines on the management of adult obesity and overweight in primary care (2002)
  An approach to weight management in children and adolescents (2–18 years) in primary care (2003)
SIGN Management of obesity in children and young people (2003)
 www.sign.ac.uk
Counterweight Project www.counterweight.org

Figure 4.7 BMI ready reckoner

Height in metres

Weight (kg)	1.36	1.40	1.44	1.48	1.52	1.56	1.60	1.64	1.68	1.72	1.76	1.80	1.84	1.88	1.92	1.96	2.00
125	68	64	60	57	54	51	49	46	44	42	40	39	37	35	34	33	31
123	67	63	59	56	53	51	48	46	44	42	40	38	36	35	33	32	31
121	65	62	58	55	52	50	47	45	43	41	39	37	36	34	33	31	30
119	64	61	57	54	52	49	46	44	42	41	40	38	37	35	34	32	31
117	63	60	56	53	51	48	46	44	41	40	38	36	35	33	32	30	29
115	62	59	55	53	50	47	45	43	41	39	37	35	34	33	31	30	29
113	61	58	54	52	49	46	44	42	40	38	36	35	33	32	31	29	28
111	60	57	54	51	48	46	43	41	39	38	36	34	33	31	30	29	28
109	59	56	53	50	47	45	43	41	39	37	35	34	32	31	30	28	27
107	58	55	52	49	46	44	42	40	38	36	35	33	32	30	29	28	27
105	57	54	51	48	45	43	41	39	37	35	34	32	31	30	28	27	26
103	56	53	50	47	45	42	40	38	36	35	33	32	30	29	28	27	26
101	55	52	49	46	44	42	39	38	36	34	33	31	30	29	27	26	25
99	54	51	48	45	43	41	39	37	35	33	32	31	29	28	27	26	25
97	52	49	47	44	42	40	38	36	34	33	31	30	28	27	26	25	24
95	51	48	46	43	41	39	37	35	34	32	31	29	28	27	26	25	24
93	50	47	45	42	40	38	36	35	33	31	30	29	27	26	25	24	23
91	49	46	44	42	39	37	36	34	32	31	29	28	27	26	25	24	23
89	48	45	43	41	39	37	35	33	32	30	29	27	26	25	24	23	22
87	47	44	42	40	38	36	34	32	31	29	28	27	26	25	24	23	22
85	46	43	41	39	37	35	33	32	30	29	27	26	25	24	23	22	21
83	45	42	40	38	36	34	32	31	29	28	27	26	25	23	23	22	21
81	44	41	39	37	35	33	32	30	29	27	26	25	24	23	22	21	20
79	43	40	38	36	34	32	31	29	28	27	26	24	23	22	21	21	20
77	42	39	37	35	33	32	30	29	27	26	25	24	23	22	21	20	19
75	41	38	36	34	32	31	29	28	27	25	24	23	22	21	20	20	19
73	39	37	35	33	32	30	29	27	26	25	24	23	22	21	20	19	18
71	38	36	34	32	31	29	28	26	25	24	23	22	21	20	19	18	18
69	37	35	33	32	30	28	27	26	24	23	22	21	20	20	19	18	18
67	36	34	32	31	29	28	26	25	24	23	22	20	19	18	18	17	17
65	35	33	31	30	28	27	25	24	23	22	21	20	19	18	18	17	16
63	34	32	30	29	27	26	25	23	22	21	20	19	19	18	17	16	16
61	33	31	29	28	26	25	24	23	22	21	20	19	18	17	17	16	15
59	32	30	28	27	26	24	23	22	21	20	19	18	17	17	16	15	15
57	31	29	27	26	25	23	22	21	20	19	18	17	16	16	15	15	14
55	30	28	27	25	24	23	21	20	19	19	18	17	16	16	15	14	14
53	29	27	26	24	23	22	21	20	18	18	17	16	15	15	14	14	13
51	28	26	25	23	22	21	20	19	18	17	16	16	15	14	14	13	13
49	26	25	24	22	21	20	19	18	17	17	16	15	14	14	13	13	12
47	25	24	23	21	20	19	18	17	17	16	15	15	14	13	13	12	12
45	24	23	22	21	19	18	18	17	16	15	15	14	13	13	12	12	11
43	23	22	21	20	19	18	17	16	15	15	14	13	13	12	12	11	11

Weight in kilograms

Legend:
- BMI <18.5 – underweight
- BMI 18.5–24.9 – acceptable weight
- BMI 25–29.9 – overweight
- BMI 30–39.9 – obese
- BMI ≥40 – morbid obesity

194

Figure 4.7 is reproduced from the *Oxford Handbook of General Practice*, 2nd edition, edited Simon, C., Everitt, H., and Kendrick, T., (2005), with permission of Oxford University Press.

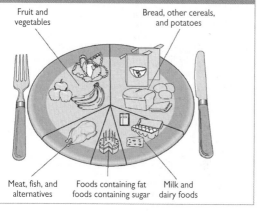

Figure 4.8 The plate model. Developed nationally to communicate current recommendations for healthy eating. It shows rough proportions of the various food groups that should make up each meal

Fruit and vegetables

Bread, other cereals, and potatoes

Meat, fish, and alternatives

Foods containing fat foods containing sugar

Milk and dairy foods

ure 4.8 is reproduced from the *Oxford Handbook of General Practice*, 2nd edition, edited by non, C., Everit, H., and Kendrick, T., (2005), with permission of Oxford University Press.

Treatment: When the body's intake is > output over a period of time, obesity results. Management of obesity aims to reverse this trend on a long-term basis.

Healthy diet: Encourage all patients to ↓ fat intake; ↑ proportion of unrefined carbohydrate; eat 5 portions of fruit and vegetables/d.; ↓ hidden sugars (alcohol, prepared foods); ↑ fibre – Figure 4.8, 📖 p.195.

Low calorie diets
- All obese people lose weight by reducing energy intake.
- A realistic goal is weight loss of 1–2lbs (0.5–1kg)/wk. and is achievable using diets of 1000–1500kcal/d. intake.
- Rates of weight loss >1kg/wk. involve loss of lean tissue rather than fat.
- Aim for a BMI of 25. There is no health benefit of weight ↓ below this.
- Weight loss in the first few weeks may be higher due to water and glycogen depletion.
- If simple diet sheets are not effective, refer to a dietician.

Very low calorie diets (<800kcal/day): Only limited place in management as this pattern of eating cannot be maintained and rebound weight gain is seen on stopping. Only use to treat morbid obesity under strict supervision.

Exercise: Regular aerobic exercise helps ↓ weight and improve health. Tailor advice to the individual and local facilities – 📖 p.198.

Drug therapy (BNF 4.5)
- Drugs specifically licensed for the treatment of obesity are orlistat (120mg tds with food) and sibutramine (10–15mg od – monitor BP and pulse rate closely).
- Consider if BMI ≥30kg/m^2 or ≥28kg/m^2 in the presence of co-morbidity e.g. DM, hypercholesterolaemia, hypertension.
- There is little evidence to guide selection but it is logical to choose orlistat for those who have a high intake of fats and sibutramine for those who cannot control their eating.
- Combination therapy involving >1 anti-obesity drug is contraindicated.

Group therapy: Group activities e.g. Weight Watchers seem to have higher success rate in producing and maintaining weight loss.

Behavioural therapy: Shown to be effective individually and in groups when combined with low calorie diets. In simplest form involves advice to avoid situations that tempt overeating.

Surgery: Only consider referral as a last resort if behavioural and dietary modification have failed and BMI >40. Gastroplasty is the most common procedure. Mortality is high.

Follow-up: On a regular basis is essential to maintain motivation.

Maintenance of weight loss: Once a patient has lost weight, diet still needs to be monitored. Ongoing follow-up has been shown to help sustain weight loss. Weight fluctuation (yo-yo dieting) may be harmful.

Use of orlistat

Warn patients about common side-effects: The major problems patients experience are GI side-effects – oily leakage from rectum, flatulence, faecal urgency, liquid or oily stools, faecal incontinence, abdominal distension and pain. GI side-effects are minimised by reduced fat intake.

NICE guidance: NICE has recommended (2001) that treatment with orlistat should be continued >6mo. only if ≥10% of starting weight has been lost since the start of treatment.

Use of sibutramine

Contraindications/cautions

- *History of psychiatric illness:* psychosis, major eating disorders, Tourette's syndrome (use with caution if family history of motor or vocal tics), drug or alcohol abuse – use with caution in depression
- *Cardiovascular disease:* avoid if history of coronary artery disease, congestive heart failure, tachycardia or other arrhythmia, peripheral arterial occlusive disease, cerebrovascular disease, uncontrolled hypertension
- *Endocrine disease:* hyperthyroidism or phaeochromocytoma
- *Prostatic hypertrophy*
- *Glaucoma:* avoid in angle closure glaucoma; use with caution if open angle glaucoma or history of ocular hypertension
- *Sleep apnoea:* use with caution – may cause ↑BP – stop if does
- *Hepatic or renal failure:* use with caution if mild – avoid if severe
- *Pregnancy or breast-feeding:* avoid
- *Epilepsy:* use with caution
- *Warfarin use or bleeding tendency:* use with caution

NICE guidance: NICE has recommended that sibutramine should be prescribed only for individuals who have attempted seriously to lose weight by diet, exercise and other behavioural modification. In addition, arrangements should exist for appropriate healthcare professionals to offer specific advice, support and counselling on diet, physical activity and behavioural strategies to those receiving sibutramine.

Monitoring: Monitor BP and pulse rate:
- every 2wk. for the first 3mo. *then*
- monthly for 3mo. *then*
- at least every 3mo.

Discontinue if blood pressure >145/90mmHg *or* if systolic or diastolic pressure raised by >10mmHg *or* if pulse rate raised by 10bpm at 2 consecutive visits.

Discontinue treatment if
- weight loss after 3mo. less than 5% of initial body weight
- weight loss stabilises at less than 5% of initial body weight
- individuals regain 3kg or more after previous weight loss

In individuals with co-morbid conditions, treatment should be continued only if weight loss is associated with other clinical benefits.

Exercise

'Lack of physical activity is a major underlying cause of death, disease and disability. Preliminary data from a WHO study on risk factors suggest that a sedentary lifestyle is one of the 10 leading global causes of death and disability. More than 2 million deaths each year are attributable to physical inactivity.'

WHO, Move for Health, 200[

In the UK, 60% of men and 70% of women are not active enough to benefit their health.

Recommended amounts of activity (DoH)
- **Adults:** ≥30min. moderate intensity exercise on ≥5d./wk.
- **Children:** ≥1h. moderate intensity exercise every day.

Dimensions of exercise
- *Volume or quantity* – quantity of activity, usually expressed as kcal per day or week. Can also be expressed as MET hours per day or week, where 1 MET = resting metabolic rate.
- *Frequency* – number of sessions per day or week.
- *Intensity* – light, moderate or vigorous. Light intensity = <4 METS (e.g. strolling), moderate = 4–6 METS (e.g. brisk walking); vigorous = 7+ METS (e.g. running).
- *Duration* – time spent on a single bout of activity.
- *Type or mode* e.g. brisk walking, dancing or weight training.

Exercise is beneficial: Regular physical activity:

↓ risk of
- CHD – physically inactive people have ~2x ↑ risk of CHD and ~3x ↑ risk of stroke[S]
- DM – through ↑ insulin sensitivity[S]
- Obesity[S] – 📖 p.192
- Osteoporosis – ↓ risk of hip fractures by ½ [S]
- Cancer – ↓ risk of colon cancer ~40%. There is also evidence of a link between exercise and ↓ risk of breast and prostate cancers[S].

Is a useful treatment for
- ↑ BP – can result in 10mmHg drop of systolic and diastolic BP. Can also delay onset of hypertension[S]
- Hypercholesterolaemia – ↑ HDL, ↓ LDL[C]
- post-MI[C] – 📖 p.72
- DM – improves insulin sensitivity and favourably affects other risk factors for DM including obesity, HDL/LDL ratio and ↑BP
- HIV – ↑ cardiopulmonary fitness and psychological well-being[C]
- Arthritis and back pain – maintains function[C]
- ↓ intensity of depression; ↓ anxiety[S].

Benefits the elderly
- Maintains functional capacity
- ↓ levels of disability
- ↓ risk of falls & hip fracture
- Improves quality of sleep[C].

Effective interventions

* *Healthcare:* ↑ physical activity for 1° and 2° prevention is effective in the short term – no evidence effects are maintained long-term. Counselling for physical activity is as effective as more structured exercise sessions.
* *Workplace:* Interventions to ↑ rates of walking to work are effective.
* *Schools:* Appropriately designed and delivered PE curricula can enhance physical activity levels. A whole school approach to physical activity promotion is effective.
* *Transport:* Well-designed interventions ↑ walking and cycling to work.
* *Communities:* Community-wide approaches to physical activity promotion → ↑ activity.

Negotiating change: It is possible to encourage people to ↑ activity levels. As with all lifestyle interventions the patient must want to change.
* If exercise levels are satisfactory, congratulate and inform about the benefits of exercise.
* If levels are unsatisfactory, explain the benefits of a higher level of physical activity and support with health education leaflets.
* Once the patient has agreed, advise and agree ways to do that.

You are more likely to be successful if:
* Exercise recommended is moderate, does not require attendance at a special facility and can be incorporated into daily life routines e.g. walking/cycling to work
* You suggest a graduated programme of exercise for sedentary patients (there is an ↑ risk of sudden cardiac death associated with sudden vigorous exercise).

Exercise schemes

* *Specialist rehabilitation schemes* (e.g. cardiac, respiratory) are in operation in many areas. They are usually operated in association with specialist services and incorporate exercise and education for patients with specific conditions e.g. post-MI (📖 p.72).
* *Exercise prescription schemes:* Collaboration between community medical services and local sports facilities. They offer low cost, supervised exercise for patients who might otherwise find it unacceptable to visit a gym, and are accessed via GP 'prescription'.
* *Local sports centres:* Many sports facilities also offer special sessions both on dry land and in the swimming pool for pregnant women, the over 50s and people with disability.

Further information

DoH National Quality Assurance Framework on Exercise Referral Systems (2001) 🖥 www.dh.gov.uk
Health Development Agency (HDA)
🖥 www.hda-online.org.uk
  Improving physical activity
  HDA guidance on the preventive aspects of the CHD NSF
  Cancer prevention: a resource to support local action in delivering the Cancer Plan
NICE Four commonly used methods to increase physical activity: brief interventions in primary care, exercise referral schemes, pedometers and community-based exercise programmes for walking and cycling (2006) 🖥 www.nice.org.uk

Alcohol misuse

Assessing drinking

Suspicious signs/symptoms: ↑ and uncontrolled BP; excess weight; recurrent injuries/accidents; non-specific GI complaints; back pain; poor sleep; tired all the time.

Ask: Assess amount, time of day, socially or alone, daily or in binges, blackouts, situations associated with heavy drinking. Consider using the CAGE questionnaire to assess dependence:
- Have you ever felt you should **C**ut down on your drinking?
- Have people **A**nnoyed you by criticising your drinking?
- Have you ever felt bad or **G**uilty about your drinking?
- Have you ever had a drink first thing in the morning to steady your nerves or to get rid of a hangover (**E**ye opener)?

Risk factors
- Previous history
- Family history
- Poor social support
- Work absenteeism
- Emotional and/or family problems
- Financial and legal problems
- Drug problems
- Alcohol associated with work e.g. publican

Examination: Smell of alcohol; tremor; sweating; slurring of speech; BP (↑ BP); signs of liver damage.

Investigations: FBC (↑ MCV); LFTs (↑ GGT identifies ~25% of heavy drinkers in general practice; ↑ AST; ↑ bilirubin). Often incidental findings.

Health risk: Continuum – individual risk depends on other factors too (e.g. smoking, heart disease, pregnancy). Recommended safe levels of alcohol consumption are <21u/wk. for men and <14u./wk. for women. Alcohol-related health problems – Table 4.11.

Table 4.11 Health risks associated with levels of alcohol consumption		
Health risk	**Men (units/wk.)**	**Women (units/wk.)**
Low	<21	<14
Intermediate	21–50	15–35
High	>50	>35

1 unit = 8g alcohol = ½ pint of beer (if strong beer can be as much as 1.75 units), small glass of wine/sherry, 1 measure of spirits (spirit measure in Scotland is 1.2 units).

1 bottle of 12% wine = 9 units.

Beneficial effects of alcohol: Moderate consumption (1–3u./d. ↓ risk of non-haemorrhagic stroke, angina pectoris and MI.

Advice for patients

Drinkline (government-sponsored helpline) ☎ 0800 917 8282
Alcohol Concern 🖥 www.alcoholconcern.org.uk
Alcoholics Anonymous ☎ 0845 7697555
🖥 www.alcoholics-anonymous.org.uk

Table 4.12 Alcohol-related problems

Death: ~40,000 deaths/y. in the UK are directly caused by alcohol.

Social

- Marriage breakdown
- Absence from work
- Loss of work
- Social isolation
- Poverty
- Loss of shelter/home

Mental health: Anxiety, depression and/or suicidal ideas; dementia and/or Korsakoffs ± Wernicke's encephalopathy

Physical

- ↑BP
- CVA
- Sexual dysfunction
- Brain damage
- Neuropathy
- Myopathy
- Cardiomyopathy
- Infertility
- Gastritis
- Pancreatitis
- DM
- Obesity
- Fetal damage
- Haemopoietic toxicity
- Interactions with other drugs
- Fatty liver
- Hepatitis
- Cirrhosis
- Oesophageal varices ± haemorrhage
- Liver cancer
- Cancer of the mouth, larynx and oesophagus
- Breast cancer
- Nutritional deficiencies
- Back pain
- Poor sleep
- Tiredness
- Injuries due to alcohol-related activity (e.g. fights)

Further information

WHO Guide to mental and neurological health in primary care: responsible drinking guidelines
⬛ www.whoguidemhpcuk.org/downloads.asp
BMJ Addiction and dependence – II: alcohol (1997) **315** 358–360
DTB Managing the heavy drinker in primary care (2000) **38**(8) 60–64
SIGN The management of harmful drinking and alcohol dependence in primary care (2003) ⬛ www.sign.ac.uk
BJGP Anderson P Effectiveness of general practice interventions for patients with harmful alcohol consumption (1993) **43** p. 386–389

Alcohol management strategies: Figure 4.9

Patients drinking within acceptable limits: Reaffirm limits.

Non-dependent drinkers: Brief GP intervention results in ~24% reducing their drinking. Provide information about safe amounts of alcohol and harmful effects of exceeding these. If receptive to change, confirm weekly consumption using a drink diary, agree targets to ↓ consumption and negotiate follow-up.

Alcohol-dependent drinkers: Suffer withdrawal symptoms if they ↓ alcohol consumption (e.g. anxiety, fits, delirium tremens – see opposite).
● If wanting to stop drinking – refer to the community alcohol team; suggest self-help organizations e.g. Alcoholics Anonymous; involve family and friends in support.
● Detoxification in the community usually uses a reducing regimen of chlordiazepoxide over a 1wk. period (20–30mg qds on days 1 and 2; 15mg qds on days 3 and 4; 10mg qds on day 5; 10mg bd on day 6; 10mg od on day 7 then stop).
● Community detoxification is contraindicated for patients with:
  ‣ Confusion or hallucinations
  ‣ History of previously complicated withdrawal (e.g. withdrawal seizures or delirium tremens)
  ‣ Epilepsy or fits
  ‣ Malnourishment
  ‣ Severe vomiting or diarrhoea
  ‣ ↑ risk of suicide
  ‣ Poor co-operation
  ‣ Failed detoxification at home
  ‣ Uncontrollable withdrawal symptoms
  ‣ Acute physical or psychiatric illness
  ‣ Multiple substance misuse
  ‣ Poor home environment.

If ambivalent/unwilling to change: Provide information; reassess and reinform on each subsequent meeting; support the family.

Vitamin B supplements: People with chronic alcohol dependence are frequently deficient in vitamins, especially thiamine – give oral thiamine indefinitely (if severe 200–300mg/d.; if mild 10–25mg/d.)[G]. During detoxification in the community, give thiamine 200mg od for 5–7d.

Relapse: Common. Warn patients and encourage them to reattend. Be supportive and maintain contact (↓ frequency and severity of relapses[G]). Consider drugs to prevent relapse e.g. acamprosate, disulfiram (specialist initiation only).

Alcohol and driving
● *Class 1 licence:* 6mo. off driving (1y. after alcohol-related seizure or detoxification)
● *Class 2 license:* Licence revoked 1y. (3y. if alcohol dependence; 5y. if alcohol-related seizure).

The DVLA arranges assessment prior to licence restoration.

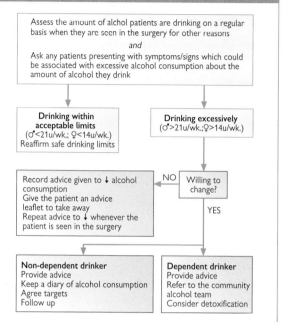

Figure 4.9 Alcohol management strategy

Assess the amount of alchol patients are drinking on a regular basis when they are seen in the surgery for other reasons

and

Ask any patients presenting with symptoms/signs which could be associated with excessive alcohol consumption about the amount of alcohol they drink

Drinking within acceptable limits
(♂<21u/wk.; ♀<14u/wk.)
Reaffirm safe drinking limits

Drinking excessively
(♂>21u/wk.; ♀>14u/wk.)

Willing to change? NO

Record advice given to ↓ alcohol consumption
Give the patient an advice leaflet to take away
Repeat advice to ↓ whenever the patient is seen in the surgery

YES

Non-dependent drinker
Provide advice
Keep a diary of alcohol consumption
Agree targets
Follow up

Dependent drinker
Provide advice
Refer to the community alcohol team
Consider detoxification

⚠ **Delirium tremens (DTs):** Major withdrawal symptoms usually occur 2–3d. after an alcoholic has stopped drinking. *Features:*
• *General:* Fever, tachycardia, ↑BP, ↑ respiratory rate
• *Psychiatric:* Vivid visual and tactile hallucinations, acute confusional state, apprehension
• *Neurological:* Tremor, fits, fluctuating level of consciousness

Action: DTs have 15% mortality and always warrant emergency hospital admission.

Chapter 5

Management of patients with chronic disability in the community

Chronic disease management

The predominant disease pattern in the developed world is one of chronic or long-term illness. In the UK, 17.5 million adults are currently living with a chronic disease. Patients with all types of heart disease, stroke, hypertension, DM and peripheral vascular disease are included in this group. Although details of chronic illness management depend on the illness, people with chronic diseases of all types have much in common with each other. *They all:*

- Have similar concerns and problems
- Must deal not only with their disease(s) but also the impact it has on their lives and emotions.

Common elements of effective chronic illness management

Involvement of the whole family: Chronic diseases do not only affect the patient but everyone in a family.

Collaboration: Between service providers and patients/carers:
- Negotiate and agree a definition of the problem
- Agree targets and goals for management
- Develop an individualized self-management plan.

Personalized written care plan: Take into account patient/carers' views and experience and the current evidence base.

Tailored education in self-management: A patient with chronic heart failure spends ~3h./y. with a health professional; the other 8757h. he manages his own condition. Helping patients with chronic disease understand and take responsibility for their condition is imperative. User-led (i.e. led by someone who suffers from the condition) self-management education programmes are most effective and are becoming increasingly available.

Planned follow-up: Pro-active follow-up according to the careplan – use of disease registers and call–recall systems is important.

Monitoring of outcome and adherence to treatment:
- Use of disease and treatment markers
- Monitoring of compliance e.g. checking prescription frequency
- Medicine management programmes

Tools and protocols for stepped care:
- Provide a framework for using limited resources to greatest effect.
- Step professional care in intensity.
- Start with limited professional input and systematic monitoring.
- Augment care for patients who do not achieve an acceptable outcome.
- Initial and subsequent treatments are selected according to evidence-based guidelines in light of a patient's progress.

Targeted use of specialist services: For those patients who cannot be managed in primary care alone.

Monitoring of process: Continually monitor management of patient with chronic disease through clinical governance mechanisms. Ensure changes are made promptly to optimize care.

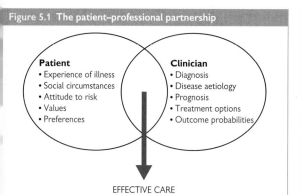

Figure 5.1 The patient–professional partnership

Patient
• Experience of illness
• Social circumstances
• Attitude to risk
• Values
• Preferences

Clinician
• Diagnosis
• Disease aetiology
• Prognosis
• Treatment options
• Outcome probabilities

EFFECTIVE CARE

GP Notes

Common patient concerns may include
- Finding and using health services
- Finding and using other community resources
- Knowing how to recognize and respond to changes in a chronic disease
- Dealing with problems and emergencies
- Making decisions about when to seek medical help
- Using medicines and treatments effectively
- Knowing how to manage stress and depression that accompany a chronic illness
- Coping with fatigue, pain and sleep problems
- Getting enough exercise
- Maintaining good nutrition
- Working with their doctor(s) and other care providers
- Talking about their illness with family and friends
- Managing work, family and social activities.

Expert patients scheme: Aims to train people with long-term chronic conditions e.g. angina, to 'self manage' their condition more effectively on a day-to-day basis.
Further Information is available at 🔲 www.expertpatients.nhs.uk

Further information
BMJ Von Korff *et al. Organising care for chronic illness* (2002) **325** p. 92–94

Rehabilitation

'Use strengthens, disuse debilitates'

Hippocrates (460–357 BC)

13–14% of the population have some disability. This is increasing as populations age and people survive longer with disability. Most patients are best managed by a multidisciplinary team in their home environment (if practicable) with a problem-oriented approach. Good interdisciplinary communication and co-ordination is essential and many patients benefit from specialist rehabilitation services. Psychological and sociocultural aspects are as important as medical aspects.

Principles of rehabilitation

- *Use of assessments/measures:* Central to management of any disability. Use validated measures accepted by all team members. Reassess regularly.
- *Teamwork:* Good outcomes are associated with clinicians working as a team towards a common goal with patients and their families (or carers) included as team members.
- *Goal setting:* Goals must be meaningful, challenging but achievable. Use short- and long-term goals. Involve the patient ± carer(s). Regularly renew, review and adapt.
- *Underlying approach to therapy:* All approaches focus on modification of impairment and improvement in function within everyday activities. Patients derive benefit from therapy focused on the management of disability.
- *Intensity/duration of therapy:* How much therapy is needed? Is there a minimum threshold below which there is no benefit at all? Studies on well-organized services show it is rare for patients to receive >2h. therapy/d. No one knows what is ideal.

Role of the GP

- The GP of any patient receiving rehabilitation in the community is a team member and may be the key worker who co-ordinates care.
- Maintain an open door policy and encourage patients and carers to seek help for problems early.
- Try to become familiar with a patient's disease, even if it is rare. It is impossible to plan care without knowledge of course and prognosis and an easy way to lose a patient's confidence if you appear ignorant of their condition.
- If progress is slower than expected, or stalls, consider other medical problems (e.g. anaemia, hypothyroidism, dementia), a neurological event, depression and communication problems (e.g. poor vision/hearing).
- Information alone can improve outcome.

Care of informal carers: 📖 p.214.

Benefits: 📖 p.225.

GP Notes: Checklist of areas to cover

- Can physical symptoms be improved?
- Can the psychological symptoms be improved (including self-esteem)?
- Can functioning within the home be improved (aids and adaptations within the home, extra help)?
- Can functioning in the community be improved (mobility outside the home, work, social activities)?
- Can the patient's or carer's financial state be improved (benefits)?
- Does the carer need more support (voluntary and self-help organizations, social services)?

Advice for patients: Information and support for patients and carers

Support organizations for the patient's condition

Department of Work and Pensions ☎ Benefits enquiry line 0800 882200; 0800 243355 (minicom facility); 0800 441144 (for help with form completion) 🖥 www.dwp.gov.uk

Citizens' Advice Bureau 🖥 www.adviceguide.org.uk

Age Concern ☎ 0800 00 99 66 🖥 www.ageconcern.org.uk

Help the Aged ☎ 0800 800 65 65 🖥 www.helptheaged.org.uk

Disabled Living Foundation: Advice about equipment and appliances ☎ 0845 130 9177 🖥 www.dlf.org.uk

Age Concern: Wide range of information and factsheets ☎ Information line 0800 00 99 66 🖥 www.ageconcern.org.uk

Royal Association for Disability and Rehabilitation (RADAR) ☎ 020 7250 3222 🖥 www.radar.org.uk

Disablement Information and Advice Line (DIAL) ☎ 01302 310123

Falls amongst the elderly

Falls are a major cause of disability and the leading cause of mortality due to injury in people aged >75y. The government sets out its strategy for tackling falls in the National Service Framework for Older People. The key interventions proposed include public health strategies to ↓ incidence of falls in the population and identification, assessment and prevention measures for those most at risk of falling.

Incidence: ↑ with age – 1:3 adults >65y. living in the community have fallen in the past year and ½ those living in institutions.

Risk factors for falls: Recurrent falls ↑ with number of risk factors:

- ♀:♂ ≈ 2:1 in the over-75s
- ↑ age
- Multiple previous falls
- Disorders of gait or balance
- Visual impairment
- Cognitive impairment
- Low morale/depression
- High level of dependence
- ↓ mobility
- Lower limb weakness or arthritis
- Foot problems
- History of stroke or Parkinson's disease
- Use of psychotropic drugs, sedatives, diuretics or β-blockers
- Alcohol
- Environmental factors (e.g. loose rugs, poor lighting, ice on the pavement, high winds)

History: Deal with the injuries first – ask about pain, loss of function, headache. Ask carers about behaviour.

Examination: Check for bruising, loss of function, confusion, BP, pulse, neurology and fundi. Consider hypothermia if on the floor any length of time.

Investigate the cause of the fall: *Consider:*

- *Physical problems:* neurological problems (e.g. stroke); visual loss; cardiac abnormalities (e.g. arrhythmia, postural hypotension); muscular abnormalities (e.g. steroid-induced myopathy); skeletal problems (e.g. osteoarthritis).
- *Environmental problems:* climbing ladders to do routine maintenance; loose/holed carpets; slippery floor or bath; chair or bed too low.

Management

- Treat any acute injury. ⓘ Subdural haematoma may take several days or weeks to reveal itself.
- Perform a falls assessment (📖 p.212) or refer to a specialist falls service for a falls assessment.
- Undertake measures to ↓ risk of falls/damage from falling.
- Specialist referral to the care-of-the-elderly team is appropriate if:
  - The cause of recurrent falls remains unclear
  - The patient or carer are worried about the possibility of further falls *or*
  - There is doubt about whether the patient can cope in their current social circumstances.

Box 5.1 Consequences of falling

- 20% who experience a fall will incur an injury requiring acute medical attention – though <1:10 falls result in a fracture (mainly Colles' and fractured neck of femur).
- Even if uninjured, older people might not be able to get up off the floor without help. The result may be a prolonged period of lying on the floor until help arrives. Apart from the indignity and helplessness this generates, secondary problems e.g. pneumonia, pressure sores, hypothermia and dehydration may follow.
- Any fall may seriously undermine an elderly person's confidence and make them (and their relatives/carers) worry about the possibility of recurrence. As a result, they may restrict activities, becoming less fit and more dependent on others.

GP Notes: Is a formal falls assessment needed?

Ask if patients fall: They may not volunteer the information spontaneously. If a patient admits to falls, or you have evidence of falls from the notes, they need a formal falls assessment.

The 'get up and go test': People who can get up from a chair without using their arms, walk several paces and return with no difficulty or unsteadiness are at low risk of falling and probably don't need a formal falls assessment.

The 'walking and talking test': People who have to stop walking while talking are at higher risk of falls and require a falls assessment.

Advice for patients: Information and support for patients and carers

Disabled Living Foundation 🖥 www.dlf.org.uk
Royal Society for the Prevention of Accidents 🖥 www.rospa.co.uk

Further information

Bandolier *Falls in the elderly*
🖥 www.jr2.ox.ac.uk/bandolier/band20/b20-5.html

Cochrane Gillespie et al. *Interventions for preventing falls in elderly people.* (2002)

British Geriatric Society Falls and Bone Health Special Interest Group 🖥 www.falls-and-bone-health.org.uk

SIGN *Prevention and management of hip fracture in older people* (2002) 🖥 www.sign.ac.uk

NICE *Guidelines for the assessment and prevention of falls* (2004). 🖥 www.nice.org.uk

BMJ Feder et al. *Guidelines for the prevention of falls in people over 65.* (2000) **321** p.1007–1011 🖥 www.bmj.com

National Service Framework for Older People 🖥 www.dh.gov.uk

Prevention of falls: Falls are one of the biggest risk factors for fracture. Tendency to fall ↑ with age. All elderly people should have their risk of falls assessed regularly – whether or not they have osteoporosis. If they are at high risk of falling, they should then have a formal falls assessment.

Falls assessment: If available, refer to a specialist falls service. *Record:*
- Frequency and history of circumstances around any previous falls
- Drug therapy: polypharmacy, hypnotics, sedatives, diuretics, antihypertensives may all cause falls
- Assessment of vision
- Examination of gait and balance, including abnormalities due to foot problems or arthritis, and motor disorders e.g. stroke
- Examination of basic neurological function, including mental status (impaired cognition and depression), muscle strength, lower extremity peripheral nerves, proprioception and reflexes
- Assessment of basic cardiovascular status, including BP (exclude postural hypotension), heart rate and rhythm
- Assessment of environmental risk factors e.g. poor lighting particularly on the stairs, loose carpets or rugs, badly fitting footwear or clothing, lack of safety equipment such as grab rails, steep stairs, slippery floors, or inaccessible lights or windows.

Measures to ↓ risk of falls and damage from falling
- Modify identified hazards or risk factors.
- Assess and correct vision, if possible.
- Correct postural hypotension – alter medication; consider compression stockings – but many elderly people cannot apply stockings tight enough to be of any use themselves.
- Treat other medical conditions e.g. refer to cardiology if arrhythmia.
- Review medication and discontinue/alter inappropriate medication.
- Remove environmental hazards – arrange bath at a day centre; refer to OT to identify and correct hazards in the home e.g. remove loose carpets, wheeled trolley for use indoors, commode or urine bottle for night time use, moving the bed downstairs etc.
- Liaise with other members of the primary healthcare team and social services to provide additional support if needed; refer to local council for 'carephone' or alarm system to call for help if any further falls.
- Refer to rehabilitation/physiotherapy to improve confidence after falls and for weight-bearing exercise (focusing on strength and flexibility) and balance training (↓ risk of falls).
- Use of hip protectors↓ fracture risk in patients at high risk but compliance is a problem[c].

General measures

- *Adequate nutrition*
  - Maintain body weight so BMI $>19 kg/m^2$.
  - Give Ca^{2+} supplements to postmenopausal women with dietary deficiency[C].
  - Supplement with Ca^{2+} (0.5–1g/d.) and vitamin D (800 IU/d.) if on long-term steroids[C], >80y., housebound or institutionalized[C].
- *Regular exercise:* Weight-bearing activity >30min/d. ↓ fracture rate[S].
- *Stop smoking*[E] Pre-menopause → 25% ↓ fracture rate postmenopause.
- ↓ *alcohol consumption* to <21u/wk. (♂) or <14u/wk. (♀).

Arrange DEXA scan to determine bone density if:

- On long-term steroids and <65y.
- Osteopoenia on X-ray
- Risk factors for osteoporosis (low BMI; FH of maternal hip fracture aged <75y.; untreated premature menopause; prolonged amenorrhoea or ♂ hypogonadism; conditions associated with prolonged immobility; medical disorder independently associated with bone loss e.g. inflammatory bowel or coeliac disease, chronic liver disease, hyperthyroidism, ankylosing spondylitis, chronic renal failure, type 1 DM, RA)
- Previous fragility fracture <75y., where non-osteoporotic causes of fracture (e.g. malignancy) have been excluded.

Treat with a bisphosphonate if

- Osteoporosis on DEXA scan
- Aged >65y. and on long-term steroids
- Aged >75y. and previous fragility fracture where non-osteoporotic causes of fracture (e.g. malignancy) have been excluded.

Care of informal carers

In the UK there are 6 million informal carers who are vitally important to the well-being of disabled people in the community. Most are relatives or friends of the person being cared for. Many are elderly with health problems themselves. There is good evidence their health suffers as a result of caring – 52% report treatment for a stress-related illness since becoming a carer and 51% report being physically injured as a result of caring.

GPs and their primary care teams are often the 1st point of access for any help needed and 88% of carers have seen their GP in the past 12 mo. Carers see the GP as the professional most able to improve their lives but few GPs have had any training about their problems and 71% carers believe their GPs are unaware of their needs.

Physical help: Record whether a patient is a carer in their notes.
- *Practical advice on nursing skills:* Ask DNs to review problems.
- *Advice on management:* Specialist nurses (e.g. CPNs etc.) provide special expertise.
- *Additional help:* Social services can provide home care. Voluntary organizations provide sitting services e.g. Crossroads schemes. Every carer has a right to ask for a full assessment of their needs by the social services.
- *Home modification:* Local authorities can arrange modifications. DNs have access to equipment needed for nursing. The Red Cross loans commodes, wheelchairs etc.
- *Respite:* Hospitals, charity organizations and local authorities provide day care (to give regular breaks each week) and respite care (for a week or more at a time).

Emotional support
- *Self-help carers' groups:* Opportunity to share experiences with people in similar situations.
- *Always ask the carer how they are when visiting* – even if they are not your patient themselves.
- *If the patient and/or carer have a religion, the clergy will often provide ongoing support.*
- *Maintain good lines of communication:* Treat the carer as a team member. Make sure you inform both carer and patient fully. Make appointments for review. Don't be short with a carer, patronising or impossible to contact.

Financial support: Many patients who have carers are entitled to Attendance Allowance or Disability Living Allowance (📕 p.234). If the patient is not expected to live >6mo. they are entitled to claim under Special Rules. This benefit is *not* means tested. Other benefits:
- *Low income* – 📕 p.230–2
- *Given up work to look after the patient* – may be eligible for Carer's Allowance – 📕 p.235
- *Substantial modification to home* – council tax may be payable at lower rate (consult local council).

GMS contract

Management indicator 9	The practice has a protocol for the identification of carers and a mechanism for the referral of carers for social services assessment	3 points

In Scotland only: Services for carers can be provided by practices as a directed enhanced service 🕮 p.261

Advice for patients: Support organizations for carers

Carers UK ☎ 020 7490 8818 🖥 www.carersuk.org
Princess Royal Trust for Carers ☎020 7480 7788
🖥 www.carers.org
Support organisations for the patient's condition
Directgov ☎ Benefits enquiry line 0800 88 22 00;
Textphone 0800 24 33 55. 🖥 www.disability.gov.uk
Citizens' Advice Bureau 🖥 www.adviceguide.org.uk
Age Concern ☎ 0800 00 99 66 🖥 www.ageconcern.org.uk
Help the Aged ☎ 0800 800 65 65 🖥 www.helptheaged.org.uk
Counsel and Care ☎ 0845 300 7585 🖥 www.counselandcare.org.uk

GP Notes: Carer skills

A carer skills course is being developed for the expert patient programe.

Further information is available at: 🖥 www.expertpatients.nhs.uk

Chapter 6

Legal aspects of care in the community

Certifying fitness to work

Own occupation test: Applies for the first 28wk. of their illness to those claiming:
- Statutory sick pay from their employer
- Incapacity benefit who have done a substantial amount of work in the 21wk. prior to the illness.

The doctor assesses whether the patient is fit to do their *own* job.

Personal capability assessment *(formerly the 'All work test')* Assesses a patient on a variety of different mental and physical health dimensions for ability to work. Not diagnosis dependent. Applies to:
- Everyone after 28wk. incapacity
- Those who do not qualify for the own occupation test from the start of their incapacity.

Claimants are sent form IB50 to complete themselves and are asked to obtain form Med 4 from their GP. If the Department of Work and Pensions (DWP) is not happy to continue paying their benefit on the basis of these reports, the applicant is called for a medical examination. Conditions relevant to mental health which exempt patients from further examination include:
- Receipt of highest rate care component of Disability Living Allowance (DLA), constant Attendance Allowance or >80% disabled for other benefit purposes
- Severe progressive cardio-respiratory disease which persistently limits exercise tolerance.

Private certificates: Some employers request private certificates in the 1st week of sickness absence. They should request it in writing. If the GP chooses to provide the service, (s)he may charge both for a private consultation and the provision of a private certificate. The company should accept full responsibility for all fees incurred by the patient.

Permitted work: Incapacity benefits do allow very limited work – therapeutic work (must be done as part of a treatment programme and in an institution which provides sheltered work for people with disabilities); voluntary work; local authority councillor; disability expert on an appeal tribunal or member of the Disability Living Allowance advisory board (not >1d./wk.).

Disability Discrimination Act 1995: In some circumstances requires employers to make reasonable adjustments for an employee with a long-term disability. Advise patients to seek specialist advice.

Disability Employment Advisors: Provided by the Employment Service to assist disabled patients to get back to work. Contacted by:
- writing a comment to the effect that intervention would be helpful in the comments box on form Med 3 *or*
- writing to the local job centre (with the patient's permission).

Table 6.1 Forms for certifying incapacity to work

Form	Use
SC1	Self-certification form for people not eligible to claim statutory sick pay who wish to claim incapacity benefit. Certifies first 7d. of illness. Available from local Jobseeker Plus offices and GP surgery.
SC2	As SC1 but for people who can claim statutory sick pay. Available from employer, local Jobseeker Plus offices and GP surgery.
Med 3	Filled in by GP or hospital doctor who knows the patient for periods of incapacity to work likely to be >7d. If return within 14d. is forecast, give fixed date of return ('closed certificate'). If longer, specify a period of time e.g. 2mo. ('open certificate'). Before the patient returns to work, reassess and give further certificate with fixed date of return. Only one Med 3 can be issued per patient per period of sickness. If mislaid, reissue and mark 'duplicate'.
Med 4	See personal capability assessment (opposite). Only completed once for any period of incapacity from work.
Med 5	Can be used if: • A doctor has not seen the patient but on the basis of a recent (<1mo.) written report from another doctor is satisfied that the patient should not work – the certificate should not cover a forward period of >1mo. • The patient returned to work without receiving a closed certificate (see Med 3 above) • >1d. since the patient was seen (so Med 3 or Med 4 cannot be issued) but it is clear the disability is ongoing.
Med 6	Used when it is felt that putting a diagnosis on a Med 3/Med 4 would be harmful either directly to a patient or through their employer knowing their diagnosis. A vague diagnosis is put on the form and a Med 6 completed which requests the Department of Works and Pensions (DWP) to send a form to obtain more precise details.
RM 7	Sent directly to the DWP to request review of the patient by them sooner than would usually be undertaken.

GP Notes: Useful information

Department of Work and Pensions *Medical evidence for Statutory Sick Pay, Statutory Maternity Pay and Social Security Incapacity Benefit purposes: a guide for registered medical practitioners.* IB204. (2004)
🖥 www.dwp.gov.uk/medical/medicalib204/ib204-june04/ib204.pdf
Disability Discrimination Act
🖥 www.direct.gov.uk/en/disabledpeople/index.htm

Fitness to drive, fly and perform other activities

Fitness to drive

> ⚠ Driving licence holders (or applicants) have a legal duty to inform the DVLA of any disability likely to cause danger to the public if they were to drive.

Driving licence types

- **Group 1:** Ordinary licence for driving a car/motorcycle. Old licences expire at 70th birthday and then must be renewed 3 yearly. Applicants are asked to confirm they have no medical disability. If so, no medical examination is necessary. New photocard licences are automatically renewed 10 yearly until age 70y. Minimum age 17y. (16y. if disabled).
- **Group 2:** Enable holders to drive lorries and buses. Min. age 21y. Initially valid until 45th birthday then renewable every 5y. until 65th birthday. >65y. renewable annually. Medical examination is needed to renew Group 2 licences. Applicants must bring form D4 (available from post offices) with them. Examinations take ~½ h. A fee may be charged by the GP.

Determining fitness to drive: Patients with any disorder which may cause danger to others if they drive should be advised not to drive and contact the DVLA. The DVLA gives advice on when they can restart.

Specific guidance regarding cardiovascular conditions: Table 6.2 📖 p.222. Unless otherwise stated, Group 1 drivers *do not* need to inform the DVLA about their condition. Group 2 drivers *always* need to inform the DVLA about their condition.

Further information

DVLA *At a glance guide to the current medical standards of fitness to drive for medical practitioners* available from 🖳 www.dvla.gov.uk

Medical advisers from the DVLA can advise on difficult issues. Contact Drivers Medical Unit, DVLA, Swansea SA99 1TU or ☎ 01792 761119

Fitness to fly: Passengers are required to tell the airline at the time of booking about any conditions that might compromise their fitness to fly. The airline's medical officer must then decide whether to carry them or not.

Hazards of flying

- Cabin pressure – oxygen levels are lower than at ground level and gas in body cavities expands 30% in flight
- Inactivity and dehydration
- Disruption of routine
- Alcohol consumption
- Stress and excitement.

Fitness to perform sporting activities: GPs are commonly asked to certify fitness to perform sports. Normally the patient will come with a medical form. If there is a form, request to see it before the medical. If there is no form and you are unsure what to check, telephone the sport's governing body or the event organizer. A fee is payable by the patient.

Many gyms and sports clubs also ask older patients and patients with pre-existing conditions or disabilities to check with their GP before they will sign them on. Assuming that a suitable regime is undertaken, most people can participate in some form of sporting activity. Consider the patient's baseline fitness, check BP and medications and recommend a gradual introduction to any new forms of exercise.

Pre-employment certification: It is becoming increasingly common for GPs to be asked about the 'medical' suitability of candidates to perform a job. This is not part of the GP's terms of service and therefore a GP can refuse to give an opinion. In all cases where an opinion is given, a fee can be claimed. Common examples are:

- Ofsted forms for childminders
- Care home staff – proof of 'physical and mental fitness'
- Food handlers – certificates of fitness.

GP Notes: What should I do if a patient continues to drive despite advice to stop?

If the patient <u>does not</u> understand the advice to stop driving: inform the DVLA.

If the patient <u>does</u> understand the advice to stop driving
- Explain your legal duty to breach confidentiality and inform the DVLA if they do not stop driving.
- If the patient still refuses to stop driving, offer a second medical opinion – on the understanding they stop driving in the interim.
- If the patient still continues driving, consider action such as recruiting next-of-kin to the cause – but beware of breach of confidentiality.
- If all else fails, write to the patient to inform him/her of your intention to inform the DVLA.
- If the patient continues to drive, inform the DVLA and write to the patient to confirm a disclosure has been made.

🚹 Always consider contacting your medical defence body for advice.

Fitness to perform certificates
⚠ Remember – signing a form may result in legal action against you should the patient NOT be fit to undertake an activity.

Where possible include a caveat e.g. 'based on information available in the medical notes the patient appears to be fit to . . . , although it is impossible to guarantee this.'

If unsure, consult your local LMC or medical defence organization for advice.

Table 6.2 DVLA guidance about fitness to drive for patients with cardiovascular problems

Condition	Group 1 licence restrictions	Group 2 licence restrictions
Angina	Stop if symptoms occur at rest or at the wheel. Restart when satisfactory symptom control is achieved.	Licence revoked if continuing symptoms (treated and/or untreated) Restored if free from angina for ≥6wk., after medical examination and exercise ECG**.
MI/Unstable angina/CABG	*After MI:* stop driving for at least 4wk. *After non-ST elevation MI:* restart driving 1wk. after successful angioplasty.	Licence revoked for at least 6wk. Renewed following medical examination and exercise ECG**.
Hypertension	Continue driving unless treatment causes unacceptable side-effects.	Licence revoked if resting BP is consistently ≥180mmHg systolic and/or ≥100mmHg diastolic. Restored if BP is controlled provided that treatment does not cause side-effects which interfere with driving.
Heart failure	Continue driving unless symptoms which distract the driver's attention.	Licence revoked if symptomatic. Restored if symptoms are controlled following medical examination and exercise ECG**, provided that the left ventricular ejection fraction is >0.4*.
Arrhythmia	Stop driving if the arrhythmia has caused or is likely to cause incapacity. Restart when the underlying cause has been identified and controlled for at least 4wk.	Licence revoked if the arrhythmia has caused or is likely to cause incapacity. Restored when the arrhythmia is controlled for at least 3mo., provided that the left ventricular ejection fraction is >0.4*.
Cardiomyopathy	Continue	Licence revoked if symptomatic. Hypertrophic cardiomyopathy: Licence restored if no more than 1 of the following criteria are not met: 1) No family history of sudden premature death from presumed HOCM. 2) Cardiologist can confirm that the HOCM is anatomically mild 3) No serious abnormality of heart rhythm. 4) Hypotension does not occur during 9min. of exercise testing.

Table 6.2 Contd.

Condition	Group 1 licence restrictions	Group 2 licence restrictions
Congenital heart disease	Continue driving. On first application/identification a report of a recent (within 2y.) examination/assessment by an appropriate consultant will be required before a licence is issued. Certain conditions require the issue of a medical review licence for 1, 2 or 3y.	Disqualifies from driving when complex or severe disorder is present. On first application/identification a recent examination/assessment by an appropriate consultant will be required before a licence is issued. Certain conditions require the issue of a medical review licence for 1, 2 or 3y.
Heart valve disease	Continue driving.	Licence revoked if symptomatic.
Single CVA/TIA/amaurosis fugax	1mo. off driving. Restart when clinically fit thereafter. Inform DVLA if residual neurological deficit 1mo. after the episode.	Licence revoked. Review after 5y.
Recurrent CVA/TIA/amaurosis fugax	Stop driving until attacks are controlled for 3mo. Inform DVLA.	Licence revoked.
Thoracic or abdominal aortic aneurysm	Inform DVLA of any aneurysm ≥6cm diameter. Driving can be continued after satisfactory medical (BP control) or surgical treatment. Stop driving if aneurysm diameter is ≥6.5cm.	Licence revoked if aneurysm diameter ≥5cm but may be restored with satisfactory medical (BP control) or surgical treatment.
Elective angioplasty	Stop driving for at least 1wk.	Licence revoked for at least 6wk. Restored if exercise test requirements can be met.
Pacemaker insertion (includes box change)	Stop driving for 1wk.	Stop driving for 6wk.
Other implantable defibrillator devices	See DVLA guidance.	See DVLA guidance.

* Left ventricular ejection fraction < 0.4 bars Group 2 entitlement.
** Exercise testing: drivers should be able to complete 3 stages of the Bruce protocol and remain free from signs of cardiovascular dysfunction, off anti-anginal medication for 48h.

Chapter 7

Benefits and support available for people with cardiac or vascular problems and their carers

Benefits

⚠ Information in this section is up to date at the time of going to press but benefits issues change rapidly.

Millions of pounds of benefits go unclaimed every year. This chapter i a rough guide to the benefits available to enable GPs to point thei patients in the right direction. It is not intended as a comprehensiv reference.

Table 7.1 Guide to agencies involved in delivering benefits to patients

Agency	Function	Website: http://www. + suffix	Telephone
Department of Work and Pensions (DWP)	Administers all benefits *except*: Tax credits (Inland Revenue) Statutory Sick Pay (employer) Housing benefit (local authority) Council tax benefit (local authorities)	dwp.gov.uk	*Benefits enquiry line:* 0800 882200 *Help with form completion:* 0800 441144 *Information for employers and the self-employed:* 0845 7143143
Jobcentre Plus	Helps people of working age to find work and get any benefits they are entitled to	jobcentreplus. gov.uk	Contact local office (list available on website)
Pension Service	Provides services and support for pensioners and people looking into pensions and retirement	thepensionservice. gov.uk	Contact area office (list available on website)
Inland Revenue	Administers tax credits	hmrc.gov.uk	Tax credit enquiry line: 0845 300 3900
Disability and Carers' Service	Delivers a range of benefits to disabled people and their carers	disability.gov.uk	Contact local disability benefits office (list available on DWP website)
Appeals Service	Provides an independent tribunal body for hearing appeals	appeals-service. gov.uk	N/A

🄳 0800 numbers are free; 0845 numbers are charged at local rate.

⚠ **Benefit fraud:** The DWP provides a freefone number which members of the public can telephone in confidence to give information about benefit fraud. ☎ 0800 85 44 40

Further information for health professionals
Department of Work and Pensions (DWP)
🖥 www.dwp. gov.uk

Further information for patients and carers
Government information and services 🖥 www.direct.gov.uk
Citizens' Advice Bureau 🖥 www.adviceguide.org.uk
Age Concern ☎ 0800 00 99 66 🖥 www.ageconcern.org.uk
Help the Aged ☎ 0800 800 65 65 🖥 www.helptheaged.org.uk
Counseland Care ☎ 0845 300 7585 🖥 www.counselandcare.org.uk

Pensions

War pensions: For people injured whilst serving in the armed forces and their dependants (if injury caused or hastened death). Administered by the Veterans Agency, MoD. No time limit for claims. *Benefits*:

War disablement pension
- *Basic benefits:* Based on percentage disablement
  - If <20% disabled – lump sum
  - If >20% disabled – weekly sum (pension)
- *Other benefits:* Allowances if severely disabled e.g.:
  - War Pensioners Mobility Supplement – for walking difficulty. Holders can apply for the motability scheme and road tax exemption
  - Constant Attendance Allowance – for high levels of care.

Medical treatment: Some services and appliances may be paid for by the Veterans Agency (includes prescription charges, nursing home fees).

Further information
Veterans Agency ☎ 0800 169 22 77 🖥 www.veteransagency.mod.uk

Retirement pension: A state retirement pension is payable to women aged ≥60y. and men aged ≥65y., even if still working. Claim forms should be received automatically – if not request one through the local Jobseeker Plus office. Pensions are taxable.

Basic pension: Flat rate amount – different for single people and married couples. If not enough National Insurance (NI) contributions have been paid amounts may ↓. >80y. higher rate payable which is not dependant on NI contributions.

Increase for dependants: Paid if:
- The claimant's spouse is <60y. and earns under a set amount/does not receive certain other benefits
- The claimant has children (if claim made before April 2003).

Additional pension: State second pension (replaced SERPS). Based on NI contributions and earnings. Workers can opt out of the additional pension scheme, pay into a private or company scheme instead and pay lower NI.

Graduated pension: Some people may be entitled to a graduated pension. This is based on earnings between 1961 and 1975.

Extra pension: For a person who defers claiming retirement pension for up to 5y. Extra pension is payable when retirement pension is claimed.

ⓘ If hospitalized, retirement pension is payable for 1y. at full rate. After 12 mo., basic pension is ↓ but additional pension stays the same.

Other benefits for pensioners
- *Pension Credit –* 📖 p.230
- *Free colour TV licence:* All pensioners >75y.
- *Winter fuel payment:* Annual payment to all pensioners >60y.
  Freephone advice service ☎0800 22 44 88

Home Responsibilities Protection (HRP): Scheme which protects basic state pension for people who don't work or have low income and are caring for someone. 🖥 www.thepensionservice.gov.uk

Christmas bonus: One-off payment made to people receiving a retirement pension or income support a few weeks before Christmas.

Cold weather payment: 📖 p.232

Table 7.2 Benefits for people with low income

	Eligibility	How to apply	Benefits gained
Income Support (IS)	• ≥18y. (16y. in some circumstances) and <60y. • Low income, <£8000 in savings (£16,000 if in residential care) and not in receipt of JSA. • <16h. paid work/wk. (and partner <24h./wk.).	Form A1 from local Jobcentre Plus office.	**Money** – depends on circumstances. **Other benefits** – housing benefit, community tax benefit, health benefits and social fund payments. Children <3y. and pregnant women – free milk and vitamins. Children >5y. – free school meals and, in some areas, uniform grants. **Christmas bonus** – 📖 p.229
JobSeekers Allowance (JSA)	• ≥19y. and <60y. (women) or <65y. (men). • Unemployed or working <16h./wk. • Capable of and available for work. • Have a JobSeekers agreement that contracts the recipient to actively seek work.	Apply by visiting local job centre.	**Contributions-based JobSeekers Allowance** – can claim for up to 26wk. Age-dependent fixed weekly payment. **Income-based JobSeekers Allowance** – allowance dependent on circumstances. Entitles claimants to same benefits as income support (see above). **Hardship payments** – Available to people disallowed JSA.
Pension credit	**Guarantee credit** – ≥60y. and income below the appropriate amount. Appropriate amount varies according to circumstances. Capital (excluding value of own home) >£6000 is deemed to count as income at the rate of £1/wk./£500 capital. **Savings credit** – ≥65y. and income > savings credit starting point – currently >£114.05/wk. for a single person or >£174.05 if one of a couple. Depends on level of income and circumstances.	Apply on form PC1. ☎ 0800 991234	**Money** – depends on circumstances. **Other benefits** – if receiving guarantee credit: automatically eligible for housing benefit, community tax benefit, and social fund payments.

Working Tax Credit (WTC)	• Age ≥16y, working ≥16h./wk. and responsible for a child (<16y. or 16–19y. in full-time education). • Age ≥16y, working ≥16h./wk. and has a disability. • Age ≥50y, working ≥16h./wk. and has started work after ≥6mo. of receiving 1 of certain benefits. • Age ≥25y. and working ≥30h./wk.	Apply to Inland Revenue. ☎ 0845 300 3900 🖥 www.hmrc.gov.uk	**Tax credits** – depends on adding together elements: • Basic element – paid to everyone entitled to WTC • Second adult element • Lone parent element • Working >30h./wk. (can combine both parents if have children) • Disability (if working >16h./wk.) • Severe disability (if working >16h./wk.) • Aged ≥50y. and in receipt of certain benefits before resuming work. • Childcare – up to 70% childcare costs.
Children's Tax Credit (CTC)	• Age ≥16y, and • Responsible for ≥1 child (<16y. or 16–19y. and in full-time education). • Family income <£50,000 pa.	Apply to Inland Revenue. ☎ 0845 300 3900 🖥 www.hmrc.gov.uk	**Tax credits:** • Family element – credit for any family eligible – if there is a child <1y. old in the family. • Child element – credit for each individual child in the family – if the child is disabled/severely disabled.
Health benefits	**Automatic entitlement:** • Age >60y. or <16y. (19y. if in full-time education). • Claiming IS or income-based JSA. • Pregnant or within 1y. of childbirth. **By application:** • Low income and • Savings <£8000.	If automatic exemption, no need to claim. If not, claim using form HC1 available from pharmacies, GP surgeries and local Jobcentre Plus offices.	Free: • Prescriptions • NHS dentistry • NHS eye tests and glasses • NHS wigs and fabric supports • Travel to hospital • Milk and vitamins for pregnant and breast-feeding women, and children <5y.

Table 7.2 Contd.

	Eligibility	How to apply	Benefits gained
Housing benefit	Low income, living in rented housing. *Exclusions:* Full-time students without dependants, people in residential care or with savings >£16,000.	Via local authority	Pays rent for up to 60wk. Then need to reapply.
Council tax benefit and second adult rebate	• **Council tax benefit** – low income. Exclusions as for housing benefit. • **Second adult rebate** – payable if someone who lives with you is aged >18y., does not pay rent or council tax and has low income. • **Council tax reduction** – if single occupier or disabled. • **Disregarded occupants** – certain people including students, carers and children are not counted in calculating the number of people living at a property.	Via local authority	**Council tax benefit** – pays council tax. **Council tax reductions:** • Single occupier – 25% discount. • All disregarded occupants – 50%. • Disabled – reduction to next lowest council tax band.
The 6 Social Fund payments	• **Crisis loan** – anyone except students and people in residential care can apply. • **Budgeting loan** – for large purchases. Must receive IS, pension credit or income-based JSA. • **Funeral payments** – must receive low income benefit and be responsible for the funeral. • **Cold weather payments** – average temperature <0°C for ≥7d. Must receive IS, pension credit or income-based JSA and live with a pensioner, child <5y. or disabled person. • **Maternity grant** • **Community care grant** – 📖 p.233	Cold weather payments – should be automatic. All others claim via local Jobcentre Plus offices or 🖥 www.dwp.gov.uk	• **Crisis loan** – up to £1000 – interest-free loan repayable when crisis finished over 78wk. • **Budgeting loan** – as crisis loan. • **Funeral expenses** – sum towards cost of funeral – usually does not cover full expenses. **Cold weather payments** – £8.50/wk.

Table 7.3 Benefits for disability and illness

	Eligibility	How to apply	Amount
Statutory Sick Pay	• Employee age ≥16y. and <65y. • Incapable of work due to sickness or disability. • Earning ≥ NI lower earnings limit. • Unable to work ≥4d. and <28wk. (inc. days when would not normally work). • Those ineligible may be eligible for Incapacity Benefit or Maternity Allowance.	Notify employer of illness – self-certification first 7d. (SC2, 📖 p.219); Med 3 after that time, 📖 p.219.	£72.55/wk. Some employers have more generous arrangements. Paid through normal pay mechanisms.
Incapacity Benefit	• Not entitled to statutory sick pay (includes self-employed). • Unable to work (Med 3 certification until Personal Capability Assessment is applied when GP may be asked for short factual report or Med 4, 📖 p.219). • < pensionable age. • Sufficient NI contributions (unless aged <20y.).	Form SC1 available from GP surgeries, hospitals and local social security offices. If employed and unable to claim SSP – apply on form SSP1 supplied by employer, ronline: www.jobcentreplus.gov.uk	1–28wk. – £61.35/wk. 29–52wk. – £72.55/wk. >52wk. – £81.35/wk. Plus additions for dependants. A higher rate is payable if <45y. when became unable to work or if over state retirement age.
Community Care Grant	Receiving Income Support or income-based Jobseeker's Allowance *and*: • want to re-establish or help the applicant or a family member stay in the community • ease exceptional pressure on the applicant or a family member. • to help with certain travel costs.	Form SF300 from local social security offices or 🖥 www.dwp.gov.uk	Minimum payment £30. No maximum amount.
Disabled Facilities Grant	For work essential to help a disabled person live an independent life. Means tested.	Apply via local housing department.	Any reasonable application for funds is considered.

Table 7.3 Contd.

	Eligibility	How to apply	Amount
Disability Living Allowance (DLA)$^\nabla$	• Disability >3mo. and expected to last >6mo. more*. • <65y. at time of application. **Mobility component:** Help needed to get about outdoors: • *Higher rate* – unable/virtually unable to walk (age >3y.). • *Lower rate* – help to find way in unfamiliar places (age >5y.). **Care component:** Help needed with personal care: • *Lower rate* – attention/supervision needed for a significant proportion of the day or unable to prepare a cooked meal. • *Middle rate* – attention/supervision throughout the day or repeated prolonged attention or watching over at night. • *Higher rate* – 24 hour attention/supervision day or terminal illness*.	☎ 0800 882200 (0800 220674 in Northern Ireland) or Leaflet DS704 available from post offices or Using claim packs available at CAB and social security offices or 🖳 www.disability.gov.uk	**Mobility component:** *Higher rate* – £45.00/wk. *Lower rate* – £17.10/wk. **Care component:** *Higher rate* – £64.50/wk. *Middle rate* – £43.15/wk. *Lower rate* – £17.10/wk.
Attendance Allowance (AA)$^\nabla$	• Disability >3mo. and expected to last >6mo. more*. • Aged ≥65y. • Not permanently in hospital or accommodation funded by the local authority. • Needs attention/supervision – higher rate if 24h. care required/terminal illness*.	☎ 0800 882200 (0800 220674 in Northern Ireland) or Leaflet DS704 available from post offices or 🖳 www.disability.gov.uk	*Lower rate* – £43.15/wk. *Higher rate* – £64.50/wk. (for people who need day *and* night care or are terminally ill).

∇ No need to receive help to apply. Not means tested.

*Terminal illness (not expected to live >6mo.) – claim under Special Rules. Claims are processed much faster and the highest care rate is automatically awarded. GP or hospital specialist fills in form DS1500 to provide clinical information to support application (fee can be claimed).

● People who need someone's help to get out of the house are entitled to free prescriptions.

Carer's Allowance	• Aged ≥16y. *and* • Spends ≥35h./wk. caring for a person with a disability who is getting AA or constant Attendance Allowance or middle or higher rate care component of DLA *and* • Earning ≤£87.00/wk. after allowable expenses. • Not in full-time education.	Complete form in leaflet DS700 available from local social security offices or 🖳 www.disability.gov.uk	£48.65/wk. *Plus additions for dependants.* (🛈 No new claims for dependent children have been accepted since April 2003.)

Table 7.4 Mobility for disabled and elderly people ● Local public transport schemes also exist.

	Eligibility	How to apply	Benefits gained
Blue Badge Scheme	Age >2y. and ≥1 of the following: War Pension Mobility Supplement Higher rate of the mobility component of DLA Motor vehicle supplied by a government health department Registered blind Severe disability in both upper limbs preventing turning of a steering wheel Permanent and substantial difficulty walking.	Apply through local social services department. ● In most circumstances the disabled person does not have to be the driver. The badge should not be used if the disabled person is not in the car. 🖥 www.dft.gov.uk	Entitles holder to park: in specified disabled spaces free of charge or time limit at parking meters or other places where waiting is limited on single yellow lines for up to 3h. (no time limit in Scotland).
Motability Scheme	Higher rate mobility component of DLA or War Pension Mobility Supplement. ● Driver may be someone else.	Contact Motability. Application guide available at 🖥 www.motability.co.uk	Registered charity. Mobility payments can be used to lease or hire-purchase a car, powered scooter or wheelchair. Grants may also be available for advance payments, adaptations or driving lessons.
Road tax exemption	Higher rate mobility component of DLA or War Pension Mobility Supplement or Person nominated as someone who regularly drives for a disabled person or Certain types of powered invalid carriages.	Usually received automatically. If not and claiming DLA ☎ 0845 7123456. If claiming War Pension ☎ 0800 1692277	Exemption from road tax.
Seatbelt exemption	Certain medical conditions e.g. colostomy	Medical practitioner must complete exemption certificate	Exemption from wearing seatbelt.

Table 7.5 Adaptations and equipment for disabled and elderly people ● **All purchases related to disability are VAT exempt.**

	Eligibility	Applying	Benefits received
Wheelchairs	Anyone requiring a wheelchair(s) for >3mo. Short-term loan of equipment is often available via the Red Cross.	Referral by GP or specialist to wheelchair service centre. Directory service centres available at 🖥 www.wheelchairmanagers.nhs.uk	Provision of suitable wheelchair. Vouchers enable disabled patients to purchase their chairs privately.
Occupational therapy (OT) assessment	All elderly or disabled people.	Request needs assessment by occupational therapist via local social services department.	Enables provision of equipment and adaptations necessary to maintain an independent lifestyle.
Disabled Living Centres/ Disability Living Foundation	All elderly or disabled people.	49 **Disabled Living Centres** in the UK – list available at 🖥 www.assist-uk.org/centres **Disabled Living Foundation** – 🖥 www.dlf.org.uk	**Disabled Living Centres** – look at and try out equipment with OTs on hand to advise. **Disabled Living Foundation** – information on aids and adaptations.
Telephone	People who have physical difficulty using the telephone or communication problems.	British Telecom produce a booklet 'Communication solutions' obtainable from ☎ 0800 800150 or 🖥 www.bt.com If difficulty using a telephone directory, register to use Directory Enquiries free ☎ 0800 5870195	Gadgets and services that make it easier for disabled or elderly people to use the telephone.
Alarm systems	Any disabled or elderly person who is alone at times, at risk, and mentally capable of using an alarm system.	Arrange via local social services or housing department. Alternatively charities for the elderly have schemes (Help the Aged – seniorlink ☎ 01255 473 999; Age Concern – Aid-Call ☎ 0800 772266).	Enables a call for help when the phone cannot be reached.

Chapter 8

The GMS contract and cardiovascular problems

The General Medical Services (GMS) contract

Although there may be some differences in process in each of the four countries of the UK, the principles of the GMS contract apply to all. A total sum for GMS services is given to each primary care organization (PCO) as part of a bigger unified budget allocation. PCOs are responsible for managing the GMS budget locally.

The contract: Made between an individual practice and a PCO. All the partners of the practice, at least one of whom must be a GP, have to sign the contract. It includes:

- National terms applicable to all practices (the 'practice contract')
- Which services will be provided by that practice i.e.
  - essential
  - additional–if not opted out
  - out-of-hours–if not opted out
  - enhanced–if opted in
- Level of quality of essential and additional services that the practice 'aspires' to
- Support arrangements e.g. IT, premises
- Total financial resources i.e. global sum + quality achievement payments + enhanced services payments + premises + IT + dispensing.

Essential services: All practices must undertake these services. *Include*

- *Day-to-day medical care of the practice population:* health promotion, management of minor and self-limiting illness and referral to secondary care services and other agencies as appropriate.
- *General management of patients who are terminally ill*
- *Chronic disease management*

Additional services: Services the practice will usually undertake but may 'opt out' of. If the practice opts out, the PCO takes responsibility for providing the service instead. The practice then receives a ↓ global sum payment.

Enhanced services: Commissioned by the PCO and paid for *in addition* to the global sum payment. 3 types:

- *Directed enhanced services:* services under national direction with national specifications and benchmark pricing which all PCOs must commission to cover their relevant population.
- *National enhanced services:* services with national minimum standards and benchmark pricing but not directed (i.e. PCOs do not have to provide these services).
- *Services developed locally* to meet local needs (local enhanced services) e.g. enhanced care of the homeless.

Table 8.1 Payment under the GMS contract

Payment	Explanation
The global sum	Major part of the money paid to practices. Paid monthly and intended to cover practice running costs. *Includes provision for:* • Delivery of essential services and additional/out-of-hours services if not opted out • Staff costs • Career development • Locum reimbursement (e.g. for appraisal, career development and protected time).
Aspiration payments	Advance payments to allow practices to develop services to achieve higher quality standards. Aspiration payments are made monthly alongside global sum payments and amount to ≈60% of the points achieved in the previous year (for 2005/6 this was ≈2004/5 points achieved × £124.60/points × 60% × list size/composition adjustment).
Achievement payments	Payments made for the practice's achieved number of points in the Quality and Outcomes Framework (☐ p.242) as measured at the start of the following year. Aspiration payments already received are deducted from the total i.e. payment for actual points less aspiration pay.
Payment for 'extra' services	Paid to practices that provide directed enhanced services, national enhanced services and/or local enhanced services to meet local needs.
Minimum practice income guarantee (MPIG)	Protects those practices that lost out under the redistribution effect of the new resource allocation formula. Calculated from the difference between the global sum allocation (GSA) under the new GMS contract and the global sum equivalent (GSE) – the amount the practice would have earned for providing the same service under the old GMS contract ('The Red Book'). If GSA < GSE, a correction factor (CF) will be applied as long as necessary so that GSA+CF=GSE.
Other payments	Payments for premises, IT and dispensing (dispensing practices only).

ⓘ The Carr-Hill allocation formula is a GMS resource allocation formula for allocating funds for the global sum and quality payments. The formula takes the practice population and then makes a series of adjustments based on the profile of the local community, taking account of determinants of relative practice workload and costs.

The Quality and Outcomes Framework

The Quality and Outcomes Framework (QOF) was developed specifically for the new GMS contract. Financial incentives are used to encourage high-quality care.

The domains: The GMS Quality Framework is divided into 4 domains

- Clinical
- Organizational
- Additional services
- Patient experience

See Table 8.2

Indicators: Every domain has a set of 'indicators' which relate to quality standards or guidelines that can be achieved within that domain. The indicators were developed by an expert group based on the best available evidence at the time and will be updated regularly. All data should be obtainable from practice clinical systems and Read codes have been developed to make this easier. Indicators are split into 3 types:

- *Structure* e.g. is a disease register in place?
- *Process:* e.g. is a particular measure being recorded? Is action being taken where appropriate?
- *Outcome:* e.g. how well is the condition being controlled?

Quality points: All achievement against quality indicators converts to points. Each point has a monetary value.

- *Yes/no indicators:* All points are allocated if the result is +ve and none if −ve.
- *Range of attainment:* For most of clinical indicators it is not possible to attain 100% results (even if allowed exceptions are applied) so a range of satisfactory attainment is specified. Minimum standard is 40%. Points are allocated in a linear fashion based on comparison with attainment against a maximum standard e.g. if the maximum % for an indicator is 90%, the minimum 40% and the practice achieves 60%, the practice will receive 20/50 (i.e. 2/5) of the available points.

Reporting on quality: Every year each practice must complete standard return form recording level of achievement and the evidence for that. In addition there is an annual quality review visit by the PCC. Based on these, the PCO confirms level of achievement funding attained and discusses points the practice will 'aspire' to the following year (📖 p.241). The process is confirmed in writing by the PCO and signed off by the practice. The Commission for Healthcare Audit and Inspection (or equivalents in Scotland/NI) checks PCO-wide quality against other PCOs countrywide.

The Quality Framework and the Personal Medical Services (PMS) contract: Mechanisms for quality delivery and the Quality Framework are broadly comparable for GMS and PMS practices. PMS practices can apply for aspiration payments and achievement payments in the same way as GMS practices. However, in order to reflect the local nature of the contracts, standards PMS practices are working to do not have to be the same as those contained in the National Quality Framework. Nevertheless, all standards must be: rigorous; evidence based; monitored fairly; assessed against criteria agreed between PCO and providers; and paid at appropriate and equitable rates.

Table 8.2 Calculation of points for quality framework payments

Components of total points score	Points	Way in which points are calculated
Clinical indicators	655	Achieving pre-set standards in management of:
		<table><tr><td>• Palliative care</td><td>• Dementia</td></tr><tr><td>• CHD</td><td>• Learning difficulty</td></tr><tr><td>• Heart failure</td><td></td></tr><tr><td>• AF</td><td>• Depression</td></tr><tr><td>• Stroke and TIA</td><td>• Mental health</td></tr><tr><td>• Hypertension</td><td>• COPD</td></tr><tr><td>• Hypothyroidism</td><td>• Asthma</td></tr><tr><td>• DM</td><td>• Epilepsy</td></tr><tr><td>• Chronic kidney disease</td><td>• Cancer</td></tr><tr><td>• Smoking</td><td>• Obesity</td></tr></table>
Organizational	181	Achieving pre-set standards in: • Records and information about patients • Information for patients • Education and training • Medicines management • Practice management
Additional services	36	Achieving pre-set standards in: • Cervical screening • Child health surveillance • Maternity services • Contraceptive services
Patient experience	108	Achieving pre-set standards in: • Patient survey* • Consultation length
Holistic care	20	Reflects range of achievement across clinical indicators – calculated by ranking clinical indicators in terms of proportion of points gained (1–10). Proportion of the points gained by the 3rd lowest indicator (i.e. indicator ranked 7) is the proportion of the holistic care points obtained.
Total possible	**1000**	

In 2005/6 and 2006/7 the average value of 1 point = £124.60

Exception reporting: 📖 p.251

Further information

DoH: The GMS Contract. 🖥 www.dh.gov.uk

BMA: The Blue book and supporting documents 🖥 www.bma.org.uk

*Improving Patient Questionnaire (IPQ – charge payable) – 🖥 www.cfep.co.uk or General Practice Assessment Questionnaire (GPAQ) – 🖥 www.gpaq.info

Coronary heart disease (CHD), Atrial fibrillation and stroke indicators of the quality and outcomes framework

Maximising points: In 2006/7, out of a total of 1000 points:
- 89 are available for CHD quality indicators (Table 8.3).
- 24 are available for stroke quality indicators (Table 8.4, 📖 p.247).
- 20 are available for management of patients with heart failure (Table 8.5, 📖 p.247).
- 30 are available for atrial fibrillation (AF) quality indicators (Table 8.6, 📖 p.249)

Disease register: The first CHD, heart failure, stroke and AF indicators all require practices to 'produce a register of patients' with those conditions. The practice reports the number of patients on its registers as a proportion of total list size.

Identifying patients with CHD: Many labels are used for coronary heart disease – angina, MI, chest pain, acute LVF, CCF. Additionally patients with conditions secondary to coronary heart disease e.g. AF, may qualify for the CHD register. Search drug lists for 'cardiac' drugs (e.g. GTN, aspirin, ACE inhibitors) and records for cardiac investigations (e.g. exercise ECG, Echocardiography) to find unrecorded diagnoses. It is up to the practice to decide when to include a patient.

Patients with metabolic syndrome who do *not* have active coronary heart disease should not be included on the CHD register.

Identifying patients with stroke/TIA: Many labels are used for stroke – stroke, TIA, cerebrovascular accident, cerebral bleed etc. It is up to a practice to decide when to include a patient – for example when does a dizzy spell become a TIA?

Identifying patients with Heart failure: Echocardiogram is diagnostic – though for the purposes of the indicators, presence of a diagnosis of heart failure in the patient record is sufficient for inclusion in the heart failure register. All patients diagnosed after 1.4.2006 should have been investigated to confirm diagnosis (HFI).

Identifying patients with AF: For the purposes of the indicators, presence of a diagnosis of AF is sufficient for inclusion in the AF register (AF1) if diagnosis was before 1.4.2006.

🛈 The PCO may compare reported and expected prevalence – know your inclusion and exclusion criteria and be able to justify them.

Table 8.3 Coronary heart disease (CHD) indicators

Indicator	Description	Points	Payment stages
CHD 1	The pratice can produce a register of patients with coronary heart disease	4 points	
CHD 2	% of patients with newly diagnosed angina (after 1.4.2003) who are refered for exercise testing and/or specialist assessment	up to 7 points	40–90%
CHD 5	% of patients with coronary heart disease whose notes have a record of BP in the previous 15mo.	up to 7 points	40–90%
CHD 6	% of patients with coronary heart disease in whom the last BP reading (measured in the last 15mo.) is ≤150/90	up to 19 points	40–70%
CHD 7	% of patients with coronary heart disease whose notes have a record of total cholesterol in the previous 15mo.	up to 7 points	40–90%
CHD 8	% of patients with coronary heart disease whose last measured total cholesterol (measured in the last 15mo.) is ≤5mmol/l	up to 17 points	40–70%
CHD 9	% of patients with coronary heart disease with a record in the last 15mo. that aspirin, an alternative anti-platelet therapy, or an anti-coagulant is being taken (unless a contraindication or side-effects are recorded)	up to 7 points	40–90%
CHD 10	% of patients with coronary heart disease who are currently treated with a β-blocker (unless a contraindication or side-effects are recorded)	up to 7 points	40–60%
CHD 11	% of patients with history of myocardial infarction (diagnosed after 1.4.2003) who are currently treated with an ACE inhibitor or Angiotensin II antagonist	up to 7 points	40–80%
CHD 12	% of patients with coronary heart disease who have a record of influenza immunisation in the preceding 1st September–31th March	up to 7 points	40–90%

Diagnosis

Exercise testing: CHD indicator 2 requires patients with newly diagnosed angina to be referred for exercise-testing or myocardial perfusion scanning to provide diagnostic and prognostic information and to identify patients who might benefit from further intervention. An alternative to referral for exercise-testing is referral to a specialist (cardiologist, general physician or GP with special interest) for evaluation.

CT scan/MRI: All patients with acute stroke should be assessed with CT/MRI (Stroke 2) as intracranial haemorrhage may be treatable if rapidly diagnosed (e.g. with neurosurgery or reversal of antithrombotic medication) and there is strong evidence that antiplatelet or anticoagulant therapy is effective in 2° prevention of ischaemic – but not haemorrhagic – stroke. It is not essential TIA patients have a CT/MRI scan – though can be helpful for management.

Report all those referred for a further investigation within 12mo. of being added to the stroke register, in whom a diagnosis of stroke has been made. Also include those referred up to 3mo. before being included on the stroke register.

Echo: Clinical diagnosis of heart failure is unreliable. ECG and natriuretic peptides are helpful aids to diagnosis but Echocardiogram is the gold standard investigation which all patients should have to confirm diagnosis (HF 2).

Report those patients who have had an echocardiogram or other diagnostic testing to confirm diagnosis any time from 3mo. before to 12mo. after being added to the register. Exception reporting (Box 8.1 📖 p.251) can be used for patients for whom further investigation is not possible – either because the patient is too frail to attend for examination or because echocardiogram facilities are not available locally.

ECG: ECG is diagnostic for atrial fibrillation. All patients with AF should have their diagnosis confirmed on ECG or by a specialist. Report the percentage of patients of the AF register diagnosed after 1.4.2006 who have confirmed diagnosis of AF (AF2).

Regular review: CHD indicators 5–8, and stroke indicators 5–8 require practices to review patients on the registers every 15mo. Indicators are designed to encourage practices to optimize secondary prevention measures in long-term management. There is a lot of overlap between disease indicators (e.g. hypertension targets in diabetes, stroke, blood pressure and CHD indicator sets). Thus, it will pay particularly to identify patients with >1 chronic disease, and aim to target 100% of them for control of these common factors.

Table 8.4 Stroke indicators

Indicator	Description	Points	Payment stages
Stroke 1	The practice can produce a register of patients with Stroke or TIA	2 points	
Stroke 2	% of new patients with stroke who have been refered for further investigation	up to 2 points	40–80%
Stroke 5	% of patients with TIA/stroke who have a record of blood pressure in the notes in the preceding 15mo.	up to 2 points	40–90%
Stroke 6	% of patients with a history TIA/stroke in whom the last blood pressure reading (measured in last 15mo.) is ≤150/90	up to 5 points	40–70%
Stroke 7	% of patients with TIA/stroke who have a record of total cholesterol in the last 15mo.	up to 2 points	40–90%
Stroke 8	% of patients with TIA/stroke who last measured total cholesterol (measured in last 15mo.) was ≤5mmol/l	up to 5 points	40–60%
Stroke 12	% of patients with stroke shown to be non-haemorrhagic, or history of TIA, who have a record that an antiplatelet agent (aspirin, clopidogrel, dipyridamole, or a combination), or an anti-coagulant is being taken (unless a contraindication or side-effects are recorded)	up to 4 points	40–90%
Stroke 10	% of patients with TIA/stroke who have had influenza immunisation in the preceding 1st September–31st March	up to 2 points	40–85%

Table 8.5 Heart failure indicators

Indicator	Description	Points	Payment stages
HF 1	The practice can produce a register of patients with heart failure	4 points	
HF 2	% of patients with a diagnosis of heart failure (diagnosed after 01.04.2006) which has been confirmed by an echocardiogram or by specialist assessment	6 points	40–90%
HF 3	% of patients with a current diagnosis of heart failure due to left ventricular dysfunction who are currently treated with an ACE inhibitor or Angiotensin Receptor Blocker, who can tolerate therapy and for whom there are no contraindications	10 points	40–80%

Reviews should include

Record of smoking status: Note whether and how much patients are smoking (Smoking 1). If the patient has never smoked this only needs to be recorded once since diagnosis – otherwise record smoking status at each review. In calculating the percentage, add the number who have never smoked together with the number recorded as ex-smokers and current smokers at review. This is divided by the total number or disease registers.

Where patients have been identified as smokers, offer smoking cessation advice and/or referral to the local smoke-stop service (Smoking 2). Report the percentage of current smokers offered smoking cessation advice.

Check blood pressure: Hypertension is a major risk factor for CHD and stroke. A reduction of diastolic BP of 5–6mmHg can ↓ risk of CHD by 20–25% and stroke by 35–40% in the next 5y. All patients with a history of CHD or stroke/TIA should have their BP regularly checked (CHD and Stroke 5) and patients with persistent hypertension on repeat measuring should be treated according to current guidelines. Report the percentage of patients on the CHD or stroke register with a BP recorded in the past 15mo.

For the purposes of the quality and outcomes framework, a target reduction of BP to ≤150/90 has been set (CHD and Stroke 6). Report the percentage of patients on the CHD/ stroke register with BP ≤150/90

🛈 Patients on the CHD or stroke register with hypertension also qualify for the hypertension register and blood pressure indicators.

Check serum cholesterol: There is evidence to suggest all patients with a history of CHD or stroke should be treated with a statin regardless of baseline cholesterol[S]. Aim to decrease cholesterol to <4mmol/l or by 25% – whichever is the lower figure.

Check blood lipids for all patients with a history of CHD or stroke/TIA (CHD and Stroke 7). Report the percentage of patients on the CHD or stroke register with a serum cholesterol level in the previous 15mo. For the purposes of the quality and outcomes framework, target cholesterol is ≤5mmol/l. Record the percentage of patients on the CHD or stroke register with serum cholesterol ≤5mmol/l (CHD and Stroke 8).

Screening for depression: Depression is common amongst patients with any chronic illness. Depression indicator 1 rewards screening patients with CHD and/or diabetes for depression with 2 screening questions:
1. During the last month, have you been bothered by feeling down, depressed or hopeless?
2. During the last month, have you often been bothered by having little interest or pleasure in doing anything?

A positive response to either question suggests the possibility of depression and should prompt further evaluation.

Table 8.6 Atrial fibrillation indicators

Indicator	Description	Points	Payment stages
AF1	The practice can produce a register of patients with atrial fibrillation	5	
AF2	% of patients with a diagnosis of atrial fibrillation (diagnosed after 1.4.2006) which has been confirmed with an ECG or by a specialist	up to 10	40–90%
AF3	% of patients with a diagnosis of atrial fibrillation who are currently treated with anti-coagulant or anti-platelet therapy	up to 15	40–90%

Table 8.7 Depression indicators relevant to CHD

Indicator	Description	Points	Payment stages
Depression 1	% of patients on the CHD and/or diabetes register for whom case finding for depression has been undertaken on 1 occasion in the past 15mo. using 2 standard screening questions (see opposite)	up to 8	40–90%

Table 8.8 Smoking targets for secondary prevention

Indicator	Description	Points	Payment stages
Smoking 1	% of patients with any, or any combination of the following conditions: <ul><li>CHD</li><li>hypertension</li><li>asthma</li><li>stroke or TIA</li><li>DM</li><li>COPD</li></ul> whose notes record smoking status in the previous 15mo. Except those who have never smoked where smoking status need only be recorded once since diagnosis	up to 33	40–90%
Smoking 2	% of patients with any or any combination of the conditions listed in 'smoking 1' whose notes contain a record that smoking cessation advice or referral to a specialist service, where available, has been offered within the previous 15mo.	up to 35	40–90%

Antiplatelet therapy or anticoagulation: Long-term antiplatelet therapy ↓ risk of non-fatal MI in patients with CHD by 20% and ↓ risk of further cerebrovascular events following stroke and in patients with AF. All patients who are not on anticoagulation should be taking aspirin (75mg for CHD; 75–300mg daily for stroke/TIA and AF) daily. Ensure a record is kept in the notes of patients who buy low dose aspirin OTC. Where patients are aspirin-intolerant, substitute an alternative (e.g. clopidogrel 75mg daily).

Record the percentage of patients with CHD, stroke/TIA and/or AF who have a record of a prescribed antiplatelet agent, anticoagulation or OTC aspirin within the past 15mo. (CHD 9 and Stroke 12, AF3)

β-blockers for patients with CHD: Long term β-blockade ↓ mortality and morbidity in patients with angina and after MI. Report the percentage of patients with CHD who have a record of being prescribed a β-blocker in the past 6mo. As evidence is not based on all patients with CHD, the target levels for this indicator have been set lower than for other process indicators.

ACE inhibitors for patients with history of MI: Several trials have shown ↓ mortality following MI with the use of ACE inhibitors. The Heart Outcome Prevention Evaluation (HOPE) study also showed that ACE inhibitors ↓ coronary events and progression of coronary arteriosclerosis in patients without left ventricular systolic dysfunction. Angiotensin II antagonists have a similar effect. Prescribe an ACE inhibitor for all patients who have had a MI unless there are specific contraindications.

Report the percentage of patients with a history of MI diagnosed after 1.4.2003 who have been prescribed an ACE inhibitor in the past 6mo.

ACE inhibitors for patients with heart failure:

- ACE inhibitors ↑ survival in patients with all grades of heart failure.
- Consider all patients with left ventricular systolic dysfunction for treatment with an ACE inhibitor unless there are specific contraindications.
- Evidence from trials suggests greatest benefits are achieved by treatment with maximum doses of ACE inhibitors, and that moderate doses are less effective.
- Titrate the dose of ACE inhibitors up to the maximum BNF recommended doses wherever possible.
- Check renal function prior to starting ACE inhibitors and after 2 wk. of treatment.
- Where an ACE inhibitor produces unacceptable side-effects an angiotensin II receptor antagonist is an alternative.

Report the percentage of patients on the heart failure register who have been prescribed an ACE inhibitor or Angiotensin II inhibitor in the past 6mo. (HF3).

Verification: The PCO may verify the figure provided by inspecting the computer output used to generate the figure; inspecting a sample of records of patients on the CHD or stroke register for evidence that checks have taken place; or inspecting a sample of records of patients claimed by the practice to have had smoking, BP or cholesterol checks for objective evidence of that claim.

Exception reporting: Likely to be high in this group due high level of co-morbidity within this group and the age of CHD and stroke patients. Where there has been exception reporting (Box 8.1), exceptions are subtracted from the number on the register in order to calculate the percentage.

Influenza vaccination: All patients with a history of CHD or stroke/TIA should have annual influenza vaccination in the autumn/ winter months. Report the percentage of patients on the CHD and stroke register who have an influenza vaccination recorded for the preceding winter (CHD 12 and Stroke 10).

Box 8.1 Valid exceptions

- Patients who refuse to attend review who have been invited ≥3x in the preceding 12mo. (there must be a record of this)
- Patients for whom it would not be appropriate to review the chronic disease due to particular circumstances e.g. terminal illness, extreme frailty
- Patients newly diagnosed within the practice or who have recently registered with the practice, who should have measurements made in <3mo. and delivery of clinical standards (e.g. BP or cholesterol measurement within target levels) in <9mo.
- Patients on maximum tolerated doses of medication whose levels remain sub-optimal
- Patients for whom prescribing a medication is not clinically appropriate e.g. due to allergy, another contraindication or adverse reaction
- Where a patient has not tolerated medication
- Where a patient does not agree to investigation or treatment (informed dissent), and this has been recorded in their medical records
- Where the patient has a supervening condition which makes treatment of their condition inappropriate eg cholesterol reduction where the patient has liver disease
- Where an investigative service or secondary care service is unavailable.

Hypertension indicators of the Quality and Outcomes Framework

Maximizing points: In 2006/7, out of a total of 1000 points:
- 15 points are available for recording BP of patients ≥45y.
- 83 points are available for hypertension quality indicators.

BP screening: Detecting elevated blood pressure and treating it is known to be an effective health intervention. 90% of the practice population will consult within a 5y. period. The limit to patients aged ≥45y. has been pragmatically chosen as the vast majority of patients develop hypertension after this age (records indicators 11 & 17).

Disease register: Hypertension indicator 1 requires the practice to 'produce a register of patients with established hypertension'.
- The Joint British Societies recommend drug therapy is started for all patients with sustained systolic BP ≥160mmHg or sustained diastolic blood ≥100mmHg despite lifestyle measures.
- Drug treatment is also indicated in patients with sustained systolic BPs ≥140mmHg or diastolic pressures of ≥90mmHg if target organ damage is present, there is evidence of established cardiovascular disease, diabetes or the 10y. risk of CVD is ↑.
- ↑ BP readings on 3 separate occasions confirm sustained high BP.

⚠ The PCO may compare reported and expected prevalence – know your inclusion and exclusion criteria and be able to justify them.

Regular review: Hypertension indicators 4 and 5 require practices to review patients on the hypertension register every 9mo. Indicators are designed to encourage practices to monitor BP and discourage smoking in this high-risk group. *Reviews should include:*

Smoking status: Note whether patients are smoking (Smoking 1, 📖 p.249). Report the percentage of patients on the hypertension disease register who have had their smoking status recorded at least once since diagnosis.

Where patients have been identified as smokers, offer smoking cessation advice and/or referral to the local smoke-stop service (Smoking 2, 📖 p.249). Report percentage of smokers offered smoking cessation advice ≥1x.

Hypertension monitoring: Frequency of follow-up for treated patients after adequate BP control is attained depends on many factors e.g. severity of hypertension, variability of BP, complexity of treatment regime, patient compliance and need for non-pharmacological advice.

For the purposes of the Quality Framework, it has been assumed follow-up will be undertaken at least 6-monthly with the audit standard being set at 9mo. For most patients a target of 140/85 is recommended but for the purposes of the Quality Framework a standard of <150/90 has been adopted (BP indicator 5). Different standards have been adopted for diabetic patients (Diabetes indicator 12 – 📖 p.255).

Table 8.8 Hypertension indicators

Indicator	Description	Points	Payment stages
Records 11	BP of patients aged ≥45y. is recorded in the preceding 5y. for ≥65% of patients	10	
Records 17	BP of patients aged ≥45y. is recorded in the preceding 5y. for ≥80% of patients	5	
BP 1	The practice can produce a register of patients with established hypertension	6	
BP 4	% of patients with hypertension in whom there is a record of BP in the past 9mo.	up to 20	40–90%
BP 5	% of patients with hypertension in whom the last BP (measured in the last 9mo.) is ≤150/90	up to 57	40–70%

❗ Points for monitoring and treating hypertension are also available in the CHD, stroke/TIA, diabetes and chronic kidney disease indicator sets.

Diabetes indicators relevant to cardiovascular disease

Maximizing points: In 2006/7 93 points out a total of 1000 are available for diabetes quality indicators – 81 for indicators directly relevant to cardiovascular disease management (Table 8.9).

Disease register: Diabetes indicator 1 requires the practice to 'produce a register of patients with diabetes'. The QOF does not specify how diagnosis of diabetes is made, so for the purposes of the QOF, a record of diabetes in the notes is all that is needed. As the care of children with DM is generally under specialist control, the register excludes patients <17y. The register also excludes patients with gestational diabetes. The practice reports the number of patients (≥17y.) on its diabetic register as a proportion of total list size .

Regular review: The indicators for diabetes are generally those which would be expected to be done or checked in an annual review. Diabetes indicators 2–17 and 20–22, require practices to review patients on the registers every 15mo. *Reviews should include:*

Checking weight: Weight control in overweight diabetics is associated with improved glycaemic control. Report the percentage of patients on the diabetic register who have had a body mass index recorded in the last 15 mo. (diabetes indicator 2).

Recording smoking status: Note whether and how much patients are smoking (Smoking 1, 📖 p.249). If the patient has never smoked only record once since diagnosis–otherwise record smoking status at each review. In calculating the percentage, add the number who have never smoked together with the number recorded as ex-smokers and current smokers at review. This is divided by the total number on the disease registers.

Where patients have been identified as smokers, offer smoking cessation advice and/or referral to the local smoke-stop service (Smoking 2, 📖 p.249). Report the percentage of current smokers offered smoking cessation advice.

Checking blood sugar control: HbA1c is a marker of long-term control of diabetes. Better control leads to fewer complications in both insulin-dependent and non-insulin-dependent patients with diabetes. In stable patients with diabetes measurements should be made at 6-monthly intervals. Measurement should occur more frequently if control is poor or there has been a change in therapy. For the purposes of the QOF, a standard of HbA1c in the previous 15mo. has been set (Diabetes indicator 5).

To reduce micro- and macro-vascular complications, aim to achieve HbA1c levels of 6.5–7.5%. For the purposes of the QOF, 2 targets have been set – ≤10% (Diabetes indicator 7) and ≤7.5% (Diabetes indicator 20).

Table 8.9 Diabetes indicators

Indicator	Description	Points	Payment stages
DM 19	The practice can produce a register of patients ≥17y. with DM, which specifies whether the patients has Type 1 or Type 2 diabetes	6	
DM 2	% of patients with diabetes whose notes record body mass index in the previous 15mo.	up to 3	40–90%
DM 5	% of diabetic patients who have a record of HbA_{1c} or equivalent in the previous 15mo.	up to 3	40–90%
DM 20	% of patients with a diabetes in whom the last HbA1c is ≤7.5* in the last 15mo.	up to 17	40–50%
DM 7	% of patients with diabetes in whom the last HbA1c is ≤10* in the last 15mo.	up to 11	40–90%
DM 21	% of patients with diabetes who have a record of retinal screening in the previous 15mo.	up to 5	40–90%
DM 9	% of patients with diabetes with a record of presence or absence of peripheral pulses in the previous 15mo.	up to 3	40–90%
DM 11	% of patients with diabetes who have a record of BP in the past 15mo.	up to 3	40–90%
DM12	% of patients with diabetes in whom the last BP was ≤145/85	up to 18	40–60%
DM 13	% of patients with diabetes who have a record of micro-albuminuria testing in the previous 15mo. (exception reporting for patients with proteinuria)	up to 3	40–90%
DM 22	% of patients with diabetes who have a record of estimated glomerular filtration rate (eGFR) or serum creatinine testing in the previous 15mo.	up to 3	40–90%
DM 15	% of patients with diabetes with a diagnosis of proteinuria/micro-albuminuria who are treated with ACE inhibitors (or A2 antagonists)	up to 3	25–70%
DM 16	% of patients with diabetes who have a record of total cholesterol in the previous 15mo.	up to 3	25–90%
DM 17	% of patients with diabetes whose last measured total cholesterol within the previous 15mo. was ≤5mmol/l	up to 6	25–60%

* or equivalent test/reference range depending on local laboratory

Report the percentage of diabetic patients who have had an HbA1c or equivalent in the previous 15mo., the percentage of diabetics with HbA1c ≤10% and the percentage of diabetics with HbA1c ≤7.5%.

Fructosamine may be used in some areas as an alternative to HbA1c or in some patients with haemoglobinopathies.

There may be variations in test availability and in normal ranges in different parts of the UK. If this is the case, the PCO may stipulate a different but equivalent range for this indicator.

Checking peripheral pulses: Patients with diabetes are at high risk of foot complications and peripheral vascular disease. Inspect the feet and check peripheral pulses as part of the annual review (diabetes indicator 9).

Checking blood pressure: Hypertension is a major risk factor for CHD and stroke. A reduction of diastolic BP of 5–6mmHg can ↓ risk of CHD by 20–25% and stroke by 35–40% in the next 5y. All patients with a history of diabetes should have their BP regularly checked (Diabetes indicator 11) and patients with persistent hypertension on repeat measuring should be treated according to current guidelines. Report the percentage of patients on the diabetes register with a BP recorded in the past 15mo.

For the purposes of the QOF a target reduction of BP to ≤145/85 has been set (Diabetes 12). Report the percentage of patients on the diabetes register with BP ≤145/85.

ⓘ Patients on the diabetes register with hypertension also qualify for the hypertension register and blood pressure indicators.

Checking serum cholesterol: There is evidence to suggest all patients ≥40y. with diabetes should be treated with a statin regardless of baseline cholesterol[S]. Aim to decrease cholesterol to <4mmol/l or by 25% – whichever is the lower figure.

Check blood lipids for all diabetic patients (Diabetes indicator 16). Report the percentage of patients on the diabetes register with a serum cholesterol level in the previous 15mo.

For the purposes of the QOF, target cholesterol is ≤5mmol/l. Record the percentage of patients on the diabetes register with serum cholesterol ≤5mmol/l (Diabetes indicator 17).

Screening for depression 📖 p.248

Verification: The PCO may verify the figure provided by inspecting the computer output used to generate the figure; inspecting a sample of records of patients on the diabetic register for evidence that checks have taken place; or inspecting a sample of records of patients claimed by the practice to have had smoking, BP or cholesterol checks for objective evidence of that claim.

Other relevant quality indicators

Smoking: Identification of smokers and helping them to stop smoking is recognized in several indicator sets in the QOF. As well as being included for secondary prevention (📖 p.249) practices are rewarded for recording the smoking status of all patients aged 15y. (Record 22) and providing literature and offering appropriate therapy (Information 5).

Obesity: Practices are rewarded for recording body mass index (BMI) and maintaining a register of adults (≥16y.) with a BMI ≥30 in the previous 15mo. (Obesity 1) In addition points can be earned for recording BMI in diabetic patients (Diabetes 2, 📖 p.255).

Dealing with emergencies: In general practice, emergencies can happen at any time without warning. It is essential that emergency equipment is ready and working (Management 7), and all drugs are in date (Medicines 3). It is also imperative that clinical (Education 1) and non-clinical (Education 5) staff know what to do in an emergency and their basic life support skills are up to date and refreshed at regular intervals.

Medication: It is important that the medicines the patient is receiving are clearly listed on his/her record and that record is kept up to date, notes have a clear indication of when the drug was started and what it was prescribed for (Records 9) and regular review of repeat medications is carried out particularly for patients on multiple drugs (Medicines 11 and 12).

Carers: Many patients with chronic cardiac problems and stroke are looked after by informal carers (📖 p.214). As a result of their caring role, many carers develop physical and mental health problems. Indentifying and supporting them (Management 9) can help maintain carer health and keep patients in the community longer.

Significant event audit (critical event monitoring): Recognized methodology for reflecting on important events in a practice. Practices undertaking significant event audit are eligible for quality points (Education 7 and 10). Myocardial infarction, especially in a young patient, would be a suitable topic.

Table 8.10 Other relevant indicators			
Indicator	Description	Points	Payment stages
Obesity 1	The practice can produce a register of patients aged ≥16y, with a BMI ≥30	8	
Records 9	For repeat medicines, an indication for the drug can be identified in the records (drugs added from 1.4.2004)	4	Minimum 80%
Records 22	% of patients aged >15y, whose notes record smoking status in the past 27mo., except those who have never smoked where smoking status need be recorded only once	11	40–90%
Information 5	The practice supports smokers in stopping smoking by a strategy which includes providing literature and offering appropriate therapy	2	
Education 1	There is a record of all practice-employed clinical staff attending training/updating in basic life support skills in the preceding 18mo.	4	
Education 5	There is a record of all practice-employed staff attending training/updating in basic life support skills in the preceding 36mo.	3	
Education 7	The practice has undertaken a ≥12 significant event reviews in the past 3y. which could include: • Any death occurring on the practice premises • Medication errors A significant even occurring when a patient may have been subjected to harm, had the circumstances/outcome been different	4	For 12 significant event reviews
Education 10	The practice has undertaken a minimum of 3 significant event reviews in the last year	6	
Management 7	The practice has systems in place to ensure regular and appropriate inspection, calibration, maintenance and replacement of equipment including: a defined responsible person; clear recording; systematic pre-planned schedules; reporting of faults	3	
Management 9	The practice has a protocol for the identification of carers and a mechanism for the referral of carers for social services assessment	3	
Mediciness 3	There is a system for checking the expiry dates of emergency drugs on at least an annual basis	2	
Medicines 11	A medication review is recorded in the notes in the preceding 15mo. for all patients being prescribed ≥4 repeat medicines	7	Minimum 80%
Medicines 12	A medication review is recorded in the notes in the preceding 15mo. for all patients being prescribed repeat medications	8	Minimum 80%

259

Enhanced services

Influenza and pneumococcal immunizations for at-risk groups as a directed enhanced service: This directed enhanced service aims to provide influenza and pneumococcal vaccination for the elderly and other 'at-risk' groups, including those taking immunosuppressant drugs for arthritis. Practices DO NOT have preferred provider status for this service.

Target group for influenza vaccination
- Patients aged ≥65y. at the end of the financial year
- Patients suffering from chronic respiratory disease (including asthma and neuromuscular disease e.g. stroke, MS, PD, MND), chronic heart disease, chronic liver disease, chronic renal disease, immunosuppression due to disease or treatment, or diabetes mellitus
- Patients living in long-stay residential or nursing homes or other long-stay health or social care facilities
- Carers of people with chronic disability.

Target group for pneumococcal vaccination
- Patients ≥65y. at the end of the financial year
- Patients suffering from chronic respiratory disease (including asthma) and patients with neuromuscular disease (e.g. cerebral palsy, stroke, MS, MND, PD), chronic heart disease, chronic renal disease or nephrotic syndrome, chronic liver disease (including cirrhosis), immunosuppression due to disease or treatment (including HIV infection at all stages), asplenia or severe dysfunction of the spleen (including homozygous sickle cell disease and coeliac disease), diabetes mellitus, or individuals with CSF shunts
- Children <5y. who have previously had invasive pneumococcal disease
- Patients living in long-stay residential or nursing homes or other long-stay health or social care facilities.

Qualifications to provide the service
- Practices are expected to use a call – recall system identifying those 'at-risk' through existing registers compiled for use within the Quality and Outcomes Framework.
- Practices not participating in the Quality and Outcomes Framework must compile a register to qualify to provide this enhanced service.

Targets
- No target has been set for the proportion of 'at-risk' patients given influenza or pneumococcal vaccination.
- A target of 70% has been set for influenza vaccination of patients ≥65y.; however, a fee per vaccination is payable whether or not this target is reached.
- Additional payments are available through the Quality and Outcomes Framework for vaccinating high proportions of 'at-risk' patients against influenza. This includes patients who have had a stroke/TIA.

Anticoagulation monitoring as a national enhanced service:
This service aims to provide an anticoagulation monitoring scheme in the community for patients started on therapy in secondary care.

Practices must
- Develop a register of anticoagulated patients – this must include name, date of birth, indication for and length of treatment and target INR
- Proved a call–recall system
- Educate newly diagnosed patients and provide ongoing information for established patients including provision of a patient-held booklet
- Create an individual management plan for each patient on the register
- Refer promptly to other services and relevant support agencies using local guidelines where they exist
- Review the patient's health at diagnosis and at least annually thereafter including checks for potential complications
- Keep records of the service provided including all information relating to significant events e.g. hospital admission, death and ensure these records are included in the GP record
- Provide ongoing training to staff involved
- Review the scheme annually including internal and external quality assurance for any computer-aided decision-making equipment or near-patient testing equipment used and audit of care of patients including untoward incidents.

It is a condition of participation in the scheme that practitioners will give notification within 72h. of the information becoming available to the practitioner to the PCO clinical governance lead of all emergency admissions or deaths of any patients covered by this service, where such an admission or death is or may be due to usage of the drug(s) in question or attributable to the relevant underlying medical condition.

Funding available: Fees vary according to whether the blood is taken in the practice or not, the sample is tested in the practice or not and the dose is monitored by the practice or not. There are 4 levels of payment. In addition a fee is payable per home visit.

Services for carers (Scotland only)
This service aims to improve services and support for informal carers. Practices must:
- Hold and maintain a register of informal carers
- Liaise with outside carer organizations to improve carer support and appoint a member of the practice team to act as a liaison officer

To receive payment (currently ≈ f1.150/practice) practices must provide their Health Board with a written report including details of the liaison officer and contacts with local agencies, how the register was compiled and number of carers on the register, how referrals to caring agencies are made.

Chapter 9

Useful information and contacts for GPs and patients

Useful information and contacts for GPs

General information
DIPEx patient experience database 🖳 www.dipex.org
British Heart Foundation ☎ 0845 0708 070 🖳 www.bhf.org.uk
National Electronic Library for Health 🖳 www.library.nhs.uk
American Heart Association 🖳 www.americanheart.org

Abdominal aortic aneurysm
British Heart Foundation Factfiles *Abdominal aortic aneurysms* (03/2003)
🖳 www.bhf.org.uk

AF
American College of Cardiology/American Heart Association/
European Society of Cardiology Guidelines for the management of
patients with AF (2001) 🖳 www.acc.org

NEJM Falk RH. *Atrial fibrillation* (2001) **344** p. 1067–1078

NICE The management of atrial fibrillation (2006) 🖳 www.nice.org.uk

Alcohol
DTB Managing the heavy drinker in primary care (2000) **38** (8) p. 60–64

SIGN The management of harmful drinking and alcohol dependence in
primary care (2003) 🖳 www.sign.ac.uk

WHO *Guide to mental and neurological health in primary care*
Includes guidelines, patient resources and checklist questionnaires
🖳 www.mentalneurologicalprimarycare.org

BMJ *Addiction and dependence – II: alcohol* (1997) **315** p. 358–360

BJGP Anderson P. *Effectiveness of general practice interventions for
patients with harmful alcohol consumption* (1993) **43** p. 386–389

Angina
SIGN Management of stable angina (2001) 🖳 www.sign.ac.uk

Anticoagulation
SIGN Antithrombotic therapy (1999) 🖳 www.sign.ac.uk

British Journal of Haematology Guidelines on oral anticoagulation
(3rd edition – 1999) **101** p. 374–387 🖳 www.bcshguidelines.com

British Journal of Clinical Pharmacology Oates et al. *A new regimen for
starting warfarin therapy in out-patients* (1998) **46** p. 157–161

Arrhythmia
British Heart Foundation Factfile *Palpitations: their significance and
investigation* (04/2004) 🖳 www.bhf.org.uk

NEJM Huikuri et al. *Sudden death due to cardiac arrhythmias* (2001) **34**
p. 1473–1482

NICE Implantable cardioverter defibrillators (ICDs) for the treatment
of arrhythmias (2006). 🖳 www.nice.org.uk

Bradycardia

NEJM Mangrum & DiMarco. *The evaluation and management of bradycardia* (2000) **342** p. 703–709

Cholesterol – see lipids

Chronic illness

BMJ Von Korff et al. *Organizing care for chronic illness* (2002) **325** p. 92–94 www.bmj.com

Clotting tendencies – see thrombophilia

Congenital heart disease

Journal of the Royal College of Physicians of London Hunter S. *Congenital heart disease in adolescence* (2000) **34** (2) p. 150–152

NEJM Brickner et al. Congenital heart disease in adults (2000) **342** (4) p. 256–263

Coronary heart disease (general)

DoH National Service Framework: Coronary Heart Disease (2000) www.dh.gov.uk

JBS2 Joint British Societies' guidelines on prevention of cardiovascular disease in clinical pratice (2005). *Heart* **91** (suppl.5): V1-52. Also available from www.bhsoc.org

British Hypertension Society *Cardiovascular risk prediction tables and Coronary heart disease event and stroke risk calculator* www.bhsoc.org

Cardiac rehabilitation www.cardiacrehabilitation.org.uk

Diabetes

NICE www.nice.org.uk
- Type 1 diabetes: diagnosis and management (2004)
- Management of type 2 diabetes: BP and lipids (2002)
- Type 2 diabetes: prevention and management of foot problems (2004)

Lancet MRC/BHF Heart Protection Study of simvastatin in diabetic patients (2003) **362** p. 2005–2016

Disability and benefits

Directgov www.disability.gov.uk

Department of Work and Pensions (DWP) www.dwp.gov.uk

DWP *Medical evidence for Statutory Sick Pay, Statutory Maternity Pay, and Social Security Incapacity Benefit purposes: A guide for registered medical practitioners. IB204. (2004).* www.dwp.gov.uk/medical/medicalib204/ib204-june04/ib204.pdf

Disability Discrimination Act www.direct.gov.uk/en/disabledpeople/index.htm

Jobcentre Plus www.jobcentreplus.gov.uk

Expert Patient Programme www.expertpatient.nhs.uk

Driving

DVLA *At-a-glance guide to the current medical standards of fitness to drive for medical practitioners* Available from dvla.gov.uk

Medical advisers from the DVLA can advise on difficult issues – contact: Drivers Medical Unit, DVLA, Swansea SA99 1TU or ☎ 01792 761119

Drugs

BNF 🖥 www.bnf.org

Medicines and Healthcare Products Regulatory Agency (MHRA formerly MCA) 🖥 www.mca.gov.uk/yellowcard

ECG

Hampton. *The ECG Made Easy* (2003) Churchill Livingstone
ISBN: 0443072523

Morris et al. *The ABC of Clinical Electrocardiography* (2002) BMJ Books
ISBN: 0727915363

Lancet Ashley et al. *Exercise testing in clinical medicine* (2000) **356** p. 1592–1597

Erectile dysfunction

British Heart Foundation Factfile *Drugs for erectile dysfunction* (06/2005) Available from 🖥 www.bhf.org.uk

Exercise

DoH *National Quality Assurance Framework on Exercise Referral Systems* (2001) 🖥 www.dh.gov.uk

Health Development Agency (HDA) 🖥 www.hda-online.org.uk
- *Improving physical activity*
- *HDA guidance on the preventive aspects of the CHD NSF*
- *Cancer prevention: a resource to support local action in delivering the Cancer Plan*

US Surgeon General *Report on Physical Activity and Health* 🖥 www.cdc.gov/nccdphp/sgr/sgr.htm

NICE Physical activity guidance (2006) 🖥 www.nice.org.uk

Falls in the elderly

Bandolier *Falls in the elderly* 🖥 www.jr2.ox.ac.uk/bandolier/band20/b20-5.html

Cochrane Gillespie et al. Interventions to prevent falls in elderly people (2002)

British Geriatric Society Falls and Bone Health Special Interest Group 🖥 www.falls-and-bone-health.org.uk

SIGN Prevention and management of hip fracture in older people (2002) 🖥 www.sign.ac.uk

NICE Guidelines for the assessment and prevention of falls (2004) 🖥 www.nice.org.uk

BMJ Feder et al. Guidelines for the prevention of falls in people over 6 (2000) **321** p. 1007–1011 🖥 www.bmj.com

National Service Framework for Older People 🖥 www.dh.gov.uk

GP contract

DoH *The GMS contract* 🖳 www.dh.gov.uk

BMA *The Blue Book and supporting documents*
🖳 www.bma.org.uk
* *Quality and Outcomes Framework guidance*
  🖳 www.bma.org.uk/ap.nsf/content/qualityoutcomes
* *Read codes* 🖳 www.bma.org.uk/ap.nsf/content/newreadcodes04

NHS Employers Confederation 🖳 www.nhsemployers.com

Heart failure

NICE *Chronic heart failure* (2003) 🖳 www.nice.org.uk

Davis *et al.* *ABC of Heart Failure* (2006) BMJ Books. ISBN: 0727916440

SIGN Diagnosis and treatment of heart failure due to left ventricular systolic dysfunction (1999) 🖳 www.sign.ac.uk

NEJM Digitalis Investigation Group *The effect of digoxin on mortality and morbidity in patients with heart failure* (1997) **336** p. 525–529

NEJM Consensus Trial Study Group. *Effects of enalapril on mortality in severe congestive heart failure: results of the North Scandinavian Enalapril Survival Study* (1987) **316** p. 1429–1436

Hypertension

NICE Hypertension: management of hypertension in adults in primary care (2004 and update 2006) 🖳 www.nice.org.uk

BS2 Joint British Societies' Guidelines on prevention of cardiovascular disease in clinical practice (2005). *Heart* **91** (Suppl. 5): V1–52. Also available at 🖳 www.bhsoc.org

BMJ Medical Research Council Working Party *MRC trial of treatment of mild hypertension: principal results* (1985) **291** p. 97–104

BMJ Medical Research Council Working Party *MRC trial of treatment of hypertension in older adults: principal results* (1992) **304** p. 405–412

BMJ Phillip *et al.* *Randomised, double-blind, multicentre comparison of hydrochlorothiazide, atenolol, nitrendipine, and enalapril in antihypertensive treatment* (1997) **315** p. 154–159

AMA Psaty *et al.* *Health outcomes associated with anti-hypertensive therapies used as first-line agents: a systematic review and meta-analysis* (1997) **277** p. 739–745

AMA ALLHAT. *Major outcomes in high-risk hypertensive patients randomized to ACE inhibitor or calcium channel blocker vs. diuretic* (2002) **88** p. 2981–2997

Journal of Human Hypertension The BHS Guidelines Working Party *Guidelines for management of hypertension: report of the fourth working party of the British Hypertension Society* (2004) **18** p. 138–185

Lancet Hansson *et al.* *Effects of intensive blood pressure lowering and low-dose aspirin in patients with hypertension: principal results of the Hypertension optimal treatment (HOT) randomised trial* (1998) **351** p. 1755–1762.

Lancet Dahlof et al. *Prevention of cardiovascular events with an anti-hypertensive regime of amlodipine adding perindopril as required, versus atenolol adding bendroflumethiazide as required, in the Anglo Scandinavian Cardiac Outcomes Trial – Blood Pressure Lowering Harm (Ascot – BPLA): a multicentre randomised controlled trial* (2005) **366** p. 895–906

NEJM Vasan et al. *Impact of high–normal blood pressure on the risk of cardiovascular disease* (2001) **345** p. 1291–1297

Infective endocarditis
British Heart Foundation Factfiles *Infective endocarditis* (12/2003 & 1/2004) ▣ www.bhf.org.uk

Lipids
JBS2 Joint British Societies' Guidelines on prevention of cardiovascular disease in clinical practice (2005). *Heart.* **91** (Suppl.5): V1-52

SIGN Lipids and the primary prevention of CHD (1999)
▣ www.sign.ac.uk

NICE Hyperlipidaemia: identification and management of hyperlipidaemia as part of cardiovascular risk assessment in 1° care (in development)
▣ www.nice.org.uk

JAMA Schwartz et al. *Effects of atorvastatin on early recurrent ischaemic events in acute coronary syndromes – the miracle study: a randomised controlled trial* (2001) **285** p. 1771–1781

Lancet MRC/BHF Heart Protection Study of cholesterol lowering with simvastatin of 5963 people with diabetes: a randomised placebo-controlled trial (2003) **362** p. 2005–2016

Lancet 4S Group *Randomised trial of cholesterol lowering in 4444 patients with coronary heart disease: the Scandinavian Simvastatin Survival Study (4S)* (1994) **344** p. 1383–1389

NEJM Shepherd et al. *Prevention of coronary heart disease with pravastatin in men with hypercholesterolaemia* (1995) **333** p. 1301–1306.

Lancet Sever et al. *Prevention of coronary and stroke events with atorvastatin in hypertensive patients who have average or lower than average cholesterol concentrations, in the Anglo Scandinavian Cardiac Outcomes trial – lipid-lowering Harman (ASCOT-LLA): a multicentre randomised controlled trial* (2003) **361** p. 1149–1158

MI
NICE MI: Secondary prevention (2007) ▣ www.nice.org.uk

Obesity
National Audit Office Tackling obesity in England (2001)
▣ www.nao.org.uk

NICE: ▣ www.nice.org.uk
- Obesity: the prevention, identification, assessment and management of overweight and obesity in adults and children (2006)
- Guidance on the use of sibutramine for the treatment of obesity in adults (2001)
- Orlistat for treatment of obesity in adults (2001)

National Obesity Forum: 🖳 www.nationalobesityforum.org.uk
- Guidelines on the management of adult obesity and overweight in primary care (2002)
- An approach to weight management in children and adolescents (2–18 years) in primary care (2003)

SIGN Management of obesity in children and young people (2003) 🖳 www.sign.ac.uk

Counterweight Project 🖳 www.counterweight.org

Palpitations – see arrhythmia

Peripheral vascular disease

British Heart Foundation Factfiles *Peripheral vascular disease* (09/2001) 🖳 www.bhf.org.uk

Journal of Vascular Surgery Dormandy & Rutherford. *Management of peripheral arterial disease* (2000) **31** p. S1–S296

NEJM Hiatt WR. *Medical treatment of peripheral arterial disease and claudication* (2001) **344** p. 1608–1621

Pre-eclampsia

Royal College of Obstetricians and Gynaecologists *Pre-eclampsia: study group recommendations* (2003) 🖳 www.rcog.org.uk

Action on Pre-eclampsia (APEC) Pre-eclampsia community guidelines (2004) 🖳 www.apec.org.uk

Pulmonary hypertension

British Heart Foundation Factfile *Pulmonary hypertension* (01/2003) 🖳 www.bhf.org.uk

Resuscitation

Resuscitation Council (UK) 🖳 www.resus.org.uk
- Resuscitation guidelines (2000)
- Cardiopulmonary resuscitation guidance for clinical practice and training in primary care (2001)
- The use of biphasic defibrillators and AEDs in children (revised 2003)

BMA, Royal College of Nursing and Resuscitation Council (UK) *Decisions relating to cardiopulmonary resuscitation* (2001) 🖳 www.resus.org.uk

Smoking

Clinical Evidence *Cardiovascular disorders – changing behaviour: smoking cessation* 🖳 www.library.nhs.uk

NICE 🖳 www.nice.org.uk
- Nicotine replacement therapy and buproprion for smoking cessation (2002)
- Brief interventions and referral for smoking cessation in primary care and other settings (2006)

Cochrane *Silagy et al. Nicotine replacement for smoking cessation* (2004) 🖳 www.library.nhs.uk

Thorax *Smoking cessation guidelines for health professionals: an update* (2000) **55** p. 987–990 🖳 thorax.bmjjournals.com

BMJ Russell. *Effect of GPs' advice against smoking* (1979) **2** p. 231–235

Stroke

Royal College of Physicians National clinical guidelines for stroke (2nd edition, 2004) ⌨ www.rcplondon.ac.uk

Cochrane Reviews ⌨ www.library.nhs.uk
- Stroke Unit Trialists' Collaboration *Organised inpatient (stroke unit) care for stroke* (2002)
- Wardlaw et al. *Thrombolysis for acute ischaemic stroke* (2003)

British Hypertension Society *Cardiovascular risk prediction tables and Coronary heart disease event and stroke risk calculator* ⌨ www.bhsoc.org

BMJ Bath & Lees. *ABC of arterial and venous disease: acute stroke* (2000) **320** p. 920–923 ⌨ www.bmj.com

BMJ Bath et al. *ABC of arterial and venous disease: secondary prevention of TIA and stroke* (2000) **320** p. 991–995 ⌨ www.bmj.com

Lancet Rothwell et al. *A simple score (ABCD) to identify individuals at high early risk of stroke after a transient ischaemic attack* (2005) **366** p. 29–36

Thrombophilia

British Committee for Standards in Haematology Diagnosis and management of heritable thrombophilia (2001)
⌨ www.bcshguidelines.com

Thrombosis/thromboembolic disease

RCOG ⌨ www.rcog.org.uk
- Thromboprophylaxis during pregnancy, labour and after vaginal delivery (2004)
- Thromboembolic disease in pregnancy and the puerperium (2001)

SIGN Antithrombotic therapy (1999) ⌨ www.sign.ac.uk

British Journal of Haematology Guidelines on oral anticoagulation (3rd edition – 1999) **101** p. 374–387 ⌨ www.bcshguidelines.com

Valvular heart disease

NEJM Carabello & Crawford. *Medical progress: valvular heart disease* (1997) **337** p. 32–41

Information and contacts for patients, relatives and carers

General information
DIPEx (patient experience database) 🖳 www.dipex.org

Patient UK (Patient information on a range of topics) 🖳 www.patient.co.uk

British Heart Foundation ☎ 0845 0708 070 🖳 www.bhf.org.uk

National Electronic Library for Health 🖳 www.library.nhs.uk

American Heart Association 🖳 www.americanheart.org

Hearts for Life 🖳 www.heartsforlife.co.uk

Alcohol
Drinkline (government-sponsored helpline) ☎ 0800 917 8282

Alcohol Concern 🖳 www.alcoholconcern.org.uk

Alcoholics Anonymous ☎ 0845 7697555
🖳 www.alcoholics-anonymous.org.uk

Aortic aneurysm – see peripheral vascular disease

Benefits
Benefit fraud line ☎ 0800 85 44 40

Citizens' Advice Bureau 🖳 www.adviceguide.org.uk

Department of Work and Pensions ☎ *Benefits enquiry line* – 0800 882200; 0800 243355 (minicom facility); 0800 441144 (for help with form completion) 🖳 www.dwp.gov.uk

Government information and services 🖳 www.direct.gov.uk

Inland Revenue 🖳 www.hmrc.gov.uk Tax credit enquiry line ☎ 0845 300 3900

Jobcentre Plus 🖳 www.jobcentreplus.gov.uk

Pension Service 🖳 www.thepensionservice.gov.uk

Veterans Agency ☎ 0800 169 22 77 🖳 www.veteransagency.mod.uk

Cardiomyopathy
Cardiomyopathy Association ☎ 01923 249 977
🖳 www.cardiomyopathy.org

Carers
Carers UK ☎ 0808 808 7777 🖳 www.carersuk.org

Counsel and Care ☎ 0845 300 7585 🖳 www.counselandcare.org.uk

Princess Royal Trust for Carers ☎ 020 7480 7788
🖳 www.carers.org

Disability and Carers' Service
🖳 www.direct.gov.uk/en/disabledpeople/index.htm

Childhood problems
Children's Heart Federation ☎ 0808 808 5000
🖳 www.childrens-heart-fed.org.uk

Parentline ☎ 0808 800 2222 🖳 www.parentlineplus.org.uk

Childline (24h. confidential counselling service) ☎ 0800 1111
🖳 www.childline.org

Congenital heart disease
Children's Heart Federation ☎ 0808 808 5000
🖳 www.childrens-heart-fed.org.uk

Diabetes
Diabetes UK ☎ 0845 120 2960 🖳 www.diabetes.org.uk

Disability
Disabled Living Foundation 🖳 www.dlf.org.uk

Citizens' Advice Bureau 🖳 www.adviceguide.org.uk

Royal Association for Disability and Rehabilitation (RADAR)
☎ 020 7250 3222 🖳 www.radar.org.uk

Disablement Information and Advice Line (DIAL) ☎ 01302 310123

Mobility Advice and Vehicle Information Service (MAVIS)
🖳 www.dft.gov.uk/access/mavis

Motability 🖳 www.motability.co.uk

Down's syndrome
Down's Syndrome Association ☎ 0845 230 0372
🖳 www.downs-syndrome.org.uk

Elderly
Age Concern ☎ 0800 00 99 66 🖳 www.ageconcern.org.uk

Help the Aged ☎ 0800 800 65 65 🖳 www.helptheaged.org.uk

Falls
Royal Society for the Prevention of Accidents
🖳 www.rospa.co.uk

Heart transplant
Transplant Support Network ☎ 0800 027 4490/1
🖳 www.transplantsupportnetwork.org.uk

Heart Transplant Families Together 🖳 www.htft.org.uk

Hypertension
Blood Pressure Association ☎ 020 8772 4994
🖳 www.bpassoc.org.uk

Peripheral vascular disease

Circulation Foundation ▢ www.circulationfoundation.org.uk/

Vascular Society of GB & Ireland ▢ www.vascularsociety.org.uk

Pre-eclampsia
Action on Pre-eclampsia UK Group (APEC) ☎ 020 8863 3271
▢ www.apec.org.uk

Smoking
Action on Smoking and Health (ASH) ☎020 7739 5902
▢ www.ash.org.uk

NHS smoking helpline ☎ 0800 169 0 169; pregnancy smoking helpline
☎ 0800 169 9 169 ▢ www.gosmokefree.co.uk

Quit helpline ☎ 0800 00 22 00 ▢ www.quit.org.uk

Stroke

Stroke Association ☎ 0845 30 33 100 ▢ www.stroke.org.uk

Northern Ireland Chest, Heart and Stroke Association
☎ 0845 76 97 299 ▢ www.nichsa.com

Chest, Heart and Stroke Association Scotland ▢ www.chss.org.uk

Different Strokes ☎ 0845 130 7172 ▢ www.differentstrokes.co.uk

Speakability ☎ 0808 808 9572 ▢ www.speakability.org.uk

Thrombosis
Lifeblood: the thrombosis charity ☎ 01406 381017
▢ www.thrombosis-charity.org.uk

Life support algorithms

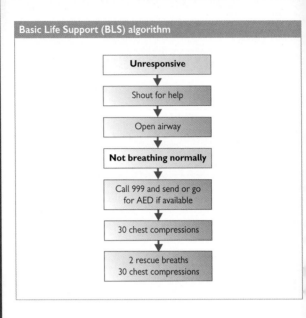

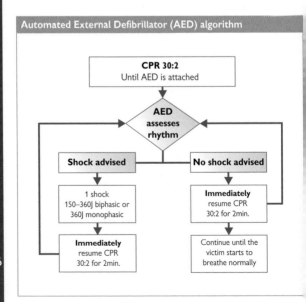

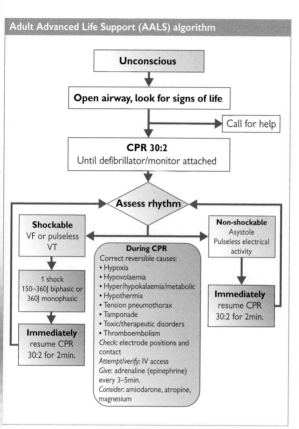

Adult Advanced Life Support (AALS) algorithm

Unconscious

Open airway, look for signs of life

→ Call for help

CPR 30:2
Until defibrillator/monitor attached

Assess rhythm

Shockable
VF or pulseless VT

1 shock
150–360J biphasic or 360J monophasic

Immediately
resume CPR 30:2 for 2min.

During CPR
Correct reversible causes:
• Hypoxia
• Hypovolaemia
• Hyper/hypokalaemia/metabolic
• Hypothermia
• Tension pneumothorax
• Tamponade
• Toxic/therapeutic disorders
• Thromboembolism
Check: electrode positions and contact
Attempt/verify: IV access
Give: adrenaline (epinephrine) every 3–5min.
Consider: amiodarone, atropine, magnesium

Non-shockable
Asystole
Pulseless electrical activity

Immediately
resume CPR 30:2 for 2min.

The Recovery Position

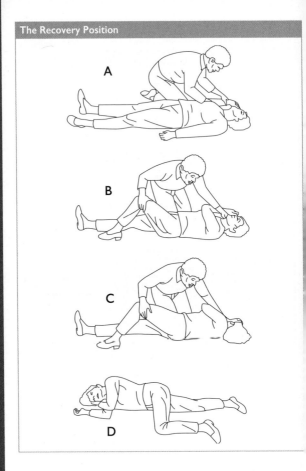

Paediatric Basic Life Support (PBLS) algorithm

Unresponsive?

↓

Shout for help

↓

Open airway

↓

Not breathing normally?

↓

5 rescue breaths

↓

Still unresponsive?
No signs of circulation

↓

15 chest compressions
2 rescue breaths

After 1 minute call for help then continue CPR

Paediatric Automated External Defibrillator (PAED) algorithm

CPR 15:2
Until AED is attached

↓

AED assesses

Shock advised

1 shock
>8y. adult shock
1–8y. paediatric attenuated

Immediately
resume CPR
15:2 for 2min.

No shock advised

Immediately
resume CPR
15:2 for 2min.

Continue until the
victim starts to
breathe normally

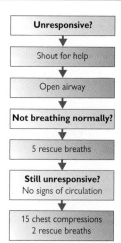
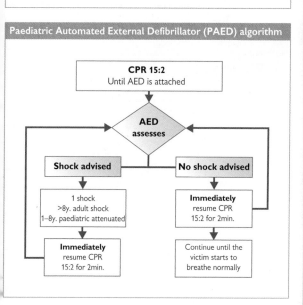

279

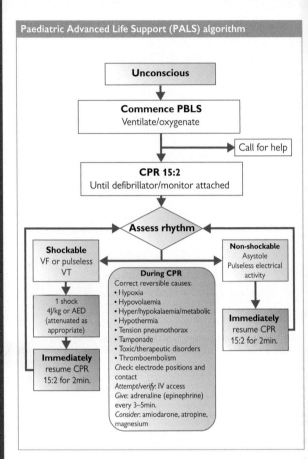

Paediatric Advanced Life Support (PALS) algorithm

Unconscious

Commence PBLS
Ventilate/oxygenate

Call for help

CPR 15:2
Until defibrillator/monitor attached

Assess rhythm

Shockable
VF or pulseless VT

1 shock
4J/kg or AED
(attenuated as appropriate)

Immediately
resume CPR
15:2 for 2min.

During CPR
Correct reversible causes:
• Hypoxia
• Hypovolaemia
• Hyper/hypokalaemia/metabolic
• Hypothermia
• Tension pneumothorax
• Tamponade
• Toxic/therapeutic disorders
• Thromboembolism
Check: electrode positions and contact
Attempt/verify: IV access
Give: adrenaline (epinephrine) every 3–5min.
Consider: amiodarone, atropine, magnesium

Non-shockable
Asystole
Pulseless electrical activity

Immediately
resume CPR
15:2 for 2min.

Index